Do's and Don'ts in
PHACO SURGERY
Text and Atlas

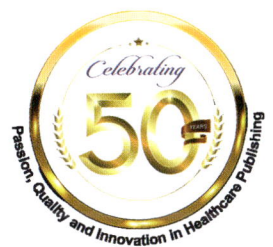

Do's and Don'ts in
PHACO SURGERY
Text and Atlas

Navneet Toshniwal
MBBS MS (Ophthalmology)
Director
Navneet Hospital
Solapur, Maharashtra, India

Forewords

Amar Agarwal
Majed Husni Al-Zoubi

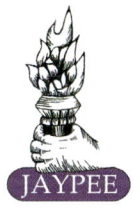

JAYPEE BROTHERS MEDICAL PUBLISHERS
The Health Sciences Publisher
New Delhi | London

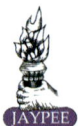 **Jaypee Brothers Medical Publishers (P) Ltd**

Headquarters
Jaypee Brothers Medical Publishers (P) Ltd.
4838/24, Ansari Road, Daryaganj
New Delhi 110 002, India
Phone: +91-11-43574357
Fax: +91-11-43574314
E-mail: jaypee@jaypeebrothers.com

Overseas Office
J.P. Medical Ltd.
83, Victoria Street, London
SW1H 0HW (UK)
Phone: +44-20 3170 8910
Fax: +44(0)20 3008 6180
E-mail: info@jpmedpub.com

Website: www.jaypeebrothers.com
Website: www.jaypeedigital.com

© 2020, Jaypee Brothers Medical Publishers

The views and opinions expressed in this book are solely those of the original contributor(s)/author(s) and do not necessarily represent those of editor(s) of the book.

All rights reserved. No part of this publication may be reproduced, stored or transmitted in any form or by any means, electronic, mechanical, photocopying, recording or otherwise, without the prior permission in writing of the publishers.

All brand names and product names used in this book are trade names, service marks, trademarks or registered trademarks of their respective owners. The publisher is not associated with any product or vendor mentioned in this book.

Medical knowledge and practice change constantly. This book is designed to provide accurate, authoritative information about the subject matter in question. However, readers are advised to check the most current information available on procedures included and check information from the manufacturer of each product to be administered, to verify the recommended dose, formula, method and duration of administration, adverse effects and contraindications. It is the responsibility of the practitioner to take all appropriate safety precautions. Neither the publisher nor the author(s)/editor(s) assume any liability for any injury and/or damage to persons or property arising from or related to use of material in this book.

This book is sold on the understanding that the publisher is not engaged in providing professional medical services. If such advice or services are required, the services of a competent medical professional should be sought.

Every effort has been made where necessary to contact holders of copyright to obtain permission to reproduce copyright material. If any have been inadvertently overlooked, the publisher will be pleased to make the necessary arrangements at the first opportunity. The **CD/DVD-ROM** (if any) provided in the sealed envelope with this book is complimentary and free of cost. **Not meant for sale**.

Inquiries for bulk sales may be solicited at: jaypee@jaypeebrothers.com

Do's and Don'ts in Phaco Surgery: Text and Atlas

First Edition: **2020**
ISBN: 978-93-89188-61-5
Printed at: Samrat Offset Pvt. Ltd.

Dedication

This book is dedicated to my Mentor and Guru Dr SS Badrinath and Dr S Vasanthi Badrinath

Blessings

Our heartiest congratulation to Dr Navneet Toshniwal on his outstanding achievement and literary contribution in the field of ophthalmology. We deeply appreciate his dedicated service in carrying forward the vision and the mission of Sankara Nethralaya in Maharashtra. Our best wishes and blessings for all his invaluable efforts and endeavors.

SS Badrinath, S Vasanthi Badrinath
President and Chairman Emeritus
Medical Research Foundation
Sankara Nethralaya
Chennai, Tamil Nadu, India

Foreword

I have been acquainted with Dr Navneet Toshniwal for more than a decade and he comes across as a great surgeon and a humble human being. He has made significant contribution towards writing books and imparting knowledge to young surgeons across the ophthalmic fraternity.

This book *Do's and Don'ts in Phaco Surgery: Text and Atlas* provides a wide variety of learning material to diversify every surgeons learning experience. The book will help create an infinite variety of thought process that the surgeons can transpose in their surgical field.

The Do's and Don'ts explained throughout the book provide a wide variety of study material and an excellent opportunity for upcoming surgeons to polish their surgical acumen. The surgeons should concentrate what they are doing and think about what they want to do before they outline their surgical line of management. The widely displayed photographs will add value to the book and I believe it will render an important tool from academic aspect.

Amar Agarwal
Chairman and Managing Director
Dr Agarwal's Group of Eye Hospitals
Chennai, Tamil Nadu, India

Foreword

It is the biggest honor for me to write foreword of this book for my best friend Dr Navneet Toshniwal.

I know Dr Navneet since 2007 when I met him first time at Dubai for MEACO conference.

I was very much impressed by his quality of Phaco work which I got chance to see him at his hospital Solapur. I invited him in July 2007 to my center Irbid, Jordan. In those days, he was the first Indian doctor who has done live Phaco surgery at Jordan.

Many times, I met him in different conferences in India and abroad and I always see him, every time he is coming with new ideas related to Phaco surgery.

He invented three instruments like Toshniwal Chopper, Toshniwal Prechopper, Toshniwal Microcapsulorhexis forcep, which I used in my practice and found to be very excellent.

I have read his two earlier books "Simplified Phacoemulsification" and "Text and Atlas: Slit Lamp Biomicroscopy for Assessment in Cataract Surgery" which are very useful and practical with great information for young doctors worldwide.

I really appreciate not only scientific view but also practical approach in his practice.

I always feel proud that true sharing of the knowledge is real quality of Dr Navneet.

This book is really masterstroke of his experiences of Phaco surgery with beautiful photographs.

Today, I really miss his father Dr Sham Toshniwal who was teacher, philosopher, friend and great human being for me.

Finally, I am feeling proud and honor to write foreword for his third book *Do's and Don'ts in Phaco Surgery: Text and Atlas*. I wish all the best for his future journey

"Go forward please"

Majed Husni Al-Zoubi MD PHD
Director
Al-Roya Eye Center
Irbid, Jordan

Preface

I have written two books earlier, from Jaypee Brothers Medical Publishers (P) Ltd., New Delhi, India. My first book *Simplified Phacoemulsification* meant for how to do surgical steps of phacoemulsification in details. The second book *Text and Atlas: Slit Lamp Bio-microscopy for Assessment of Cataract* is giving the idea of how to see cataract just before going to surgery. After writing those two books, I got confidence to give some more materials related to phacoemulsification to ophthalmic fraternity. I have started Phaco training program in 2002 under the able guidance of my father late Dr Sham Toshniwal.

One of the best points of Phaco training is analysis of surgical steps of Phaco, an analysis is depending upon the different ways of recordings, first we started with video cassettes recording (VCR), then on CDs and DVDs and now on a hard disc and a software named surgical media center (SMC). All these tools are recording the microscopic view of surgical steps, which is very significant way to guide the doctors. As the days pass, thinking of another way of analysis which consists of recording of external hand movement of surgeons. This external hand movement and microscopic view have changed the concept of Phaco training to a higher level.

In the last 6 years of this training practice, I realized that videos of surgical steps are important but in a short memory of our mind, we may forget some of the analytical points.

While watching videos we may overlook many important steps to watch. While discussing with one of the doctors during Phaco analysis, I realized that instead of videos if we take a series of photographs of that case and then discuss, I felt that photography is really one of the important ways in analysis of Phaco surgery.

Thus, in this book, I used photographs. These photographs consist pictures of surgical steps from incision to intraocular lens (IOL) implantation, handling of the instruments, correlation or coordination of instrument with particular steps, and position of eyeball.

All these points are evaluated very efficiently with these photographic pictures.

Now in my practice of this training, these photographs are most important tool for guiding doctors worldwide.

Everyone realizes or memorizes in his life that photos are better than videos of his/her events from childhood, birthday, marriage, family functions, festivals, social functions and other ceremonies and the same feeling of mine felt during this photographic way of analysis for phaco surgery.

I noticed some of the advantages such as:
- Duration of learning curve of Phaco surgery has been decreased.
- Handling of very delicate tissue has been much improved many folds.
- Understanding of the concepts of this subject was much improved.
- Doctors can get more time to think and more impact on mind with these photographs.
- Quality of analysis of Phaco surgery is better with serial of photographs than video.

I felt that putting all these classical figures or frames in the form of book will help the doctors worldwide. Such a type of book content will really help doctors who are in early and mid-phase of Phaco practice.

One of the most important aim of writing this book is that surgeons should record and analyze their own cases by photography and learn from it by themselves. The photography we have done by recording cases by Google Chrome and playing the video on VLC media player then taking screen shots. I always feel happy for sharing of my knowledge that gives me new ideas or concepts of writing such a type of book.

Navneet Toshniwal

Acknowledgments

In the journey of writing this third book, the most important motivation is appreciation and encouragement which I received from my colleague doctors not only from India but also from different parts of the world.

My first two books namely *Simplified Phacoemulsification* and *Text and Atlas*: *Slit Lamp Bio-microscopy for Assessment in Cataract Surgery* from Jaypee Brothers Medical Publishers (P) Ltd., New Delhi, India, are always great motivation to write this third book in phacoemulsification surgery.

Today, I really miss my father late Dr Sham Toshniwal who was guide, mentor, guru throughout my ophthalmology career. I even cannot attempt to write this book without his blessings. My mother Chand Toshniwal who has always taught me to give and share the knowledge to doctors and her next sentence is your knowledge will increase by sharing it in purified way.

Real Academics, I learned during my fellowship at Sankara Nethralaya, Chennai, Tamil Nadu, India, under able guidance of Dr SS Badrinath sir and Dr Vasanthi Badrinath. This is great motivation for me always. My mentor Dr Amar Agarwal who has really encouraged me in my career especially in cataract training program. I am really thankful, honored and obliged to Dr Amar Agarwal for writing foreword of this book. My sincere thanks to Dr TP Lahane sir, Dr Ragini Parekh, Dr Nitin, Dr Medha Prabudesai, Dr Pramod and Muna Bhende for encouragement and supporting me for this work. I am also thankful to Dr Majed Husni Al-Zoubi from Irbid, Jordan who has helped and encouraged me throughout in my career and honored to write foreword. I always get support and best wishes from all members of Solapur Ophthalmological Society. I am deeply indebted to brother Dr Nitin and Dr Kirti Toshniwal, sister, Dr Neeta and Dr Nilesh Bhandari, uncle Dr Murali Toshniwal who has encouraged and motivated me throughout this journey. My wife Sunita was a real backbone and support to me as usual. My mentor Ramkisanji Mundada, maternal uncle Suresh Inani, My uncle Babulalji, Mukund Toshniwal and all Toshniwal family members supported me for this work.

In completion of this book Dr Yazan Zahran (Saudi Arabia), Dr Michael Mimouni (Israel), Dr Mohammed Fouad (Egypt) Optometrist Mr. Nilesh Pundkar and Mr. Yogesh Mundhe has taken lot of efforts for this book.

My elder son Dr Nikhil who is doing MS Ophthalmology at DY Patil Medical College, Pune, Maharashtra, my younger son Sumit and nephew

Amit who is studying in third year MBBS at MRMC, Gulbarga, Karnataka have also helped a lot for editing of this book.

My special thanks to Mr Jitendar P Vij (Group Chairman), Mr Ankit Vij (Managing Director), Mr MS Mani (Group President), Ms Chetna Malhotra Vohra (Associate Director—Content Strategy), Ms Pooja Bhandari (Production Head), Ruby Sharma, Nikita Chauhan (Development Editor), and all concerned team members of M/S Jaypee Brothers Medical Publishers (P) Ltd. New Delhi, India for helping me for this book.

Thanks to Kamlesh Akude and all team of Navneet Hospital, Solapur, Maharashtra, India.

Last but not least, I would like my real thank and gratitude toward all patients, as without them we could not do this noble profession.

Contents

1. Incision 1
2. Capsulorhexis 15
3. Hydroprocedures 44
4. Trench 52
5. Division of Nucleus 68
6. Hold and Chop of Nucleus 98
7. Removal of Pieces of Nucleus 131
8. Irrigation - Aspiration of Epinucleus and Cortex 145
9. Intraocular Lens Implantation 163
10. Surgical Media Center 180

Index 189

CHAPTER 1

Incision

INTRODUCTION

- First important step of phaco surgery.
- Excellent incision architecture is important for phaco fluidics.
- Quality of incision depends on use of good blades.
- Instruments used are keratome blade, 15 degree blade, curved 19G or 20G MVR blade, crescent, and 15 no. blade.

KERATOME

Observation (Figs. 1A and B)

Air bubble is obscuring visualization of keratome entry.

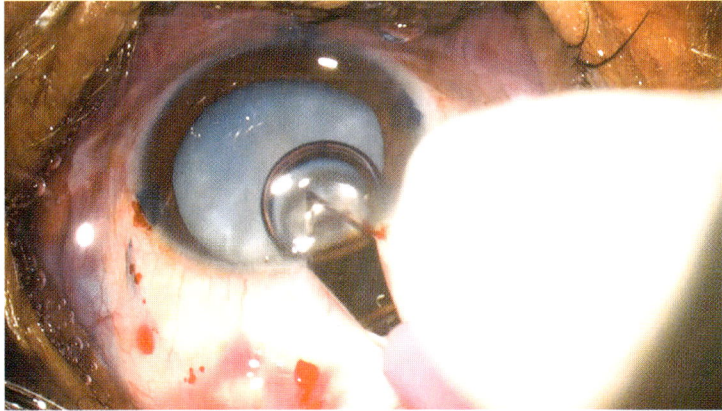

Fig. 1.1A

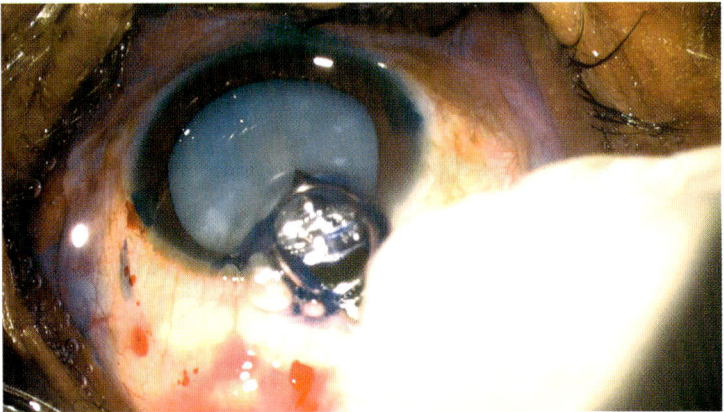

Fig. 1B

Results

- Injury to cornea can occur.
- Injury to anterior capsule can occur.

Do's
- Air bubble is often present in anterior chamber.
- With keratome entry air bubble comes out, for further smooth entry.

Observations (Figs. 2A to C)

- Fingers are seen in the microscopic view during incision.
- Placement of fingers near the tip of keratome.

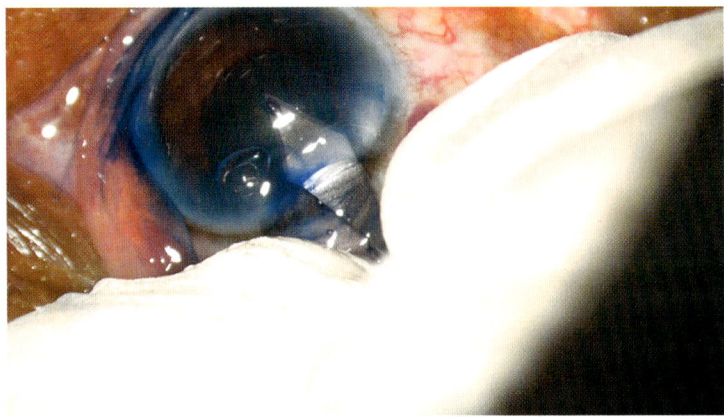

Fig. 2A

Incision

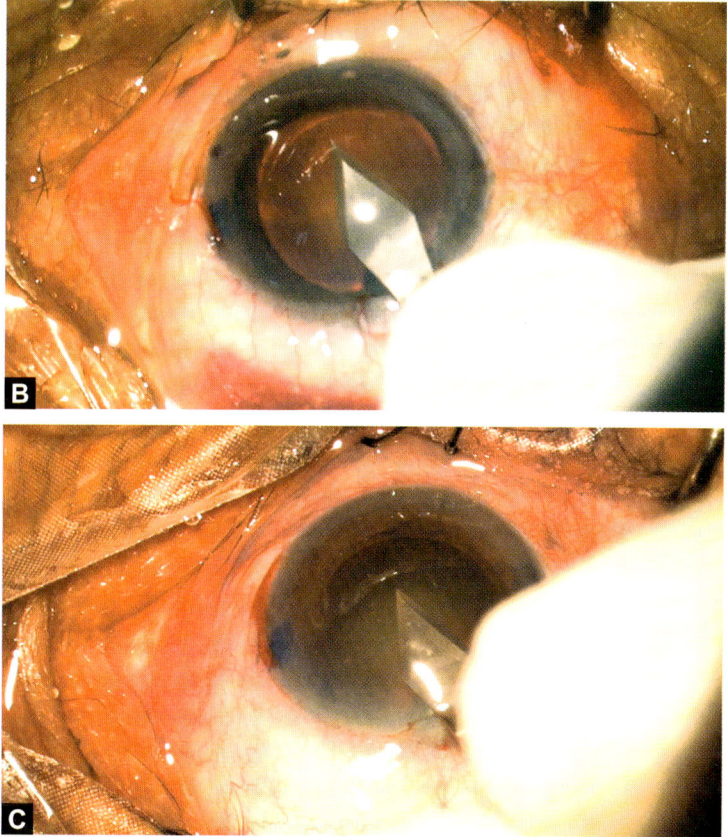

Figs. 2B and C

Results

- More pressure during keratome entry can cause injury to anterior capsule.
- Eyeball can move inferiorly which makes procedure difficult.

Do's
One should hold keratome at proper site of handle, i.e. away from the tip of keratome.

Observation (Figs. 3A and B)

Folds on cornea seen during keratome entry.

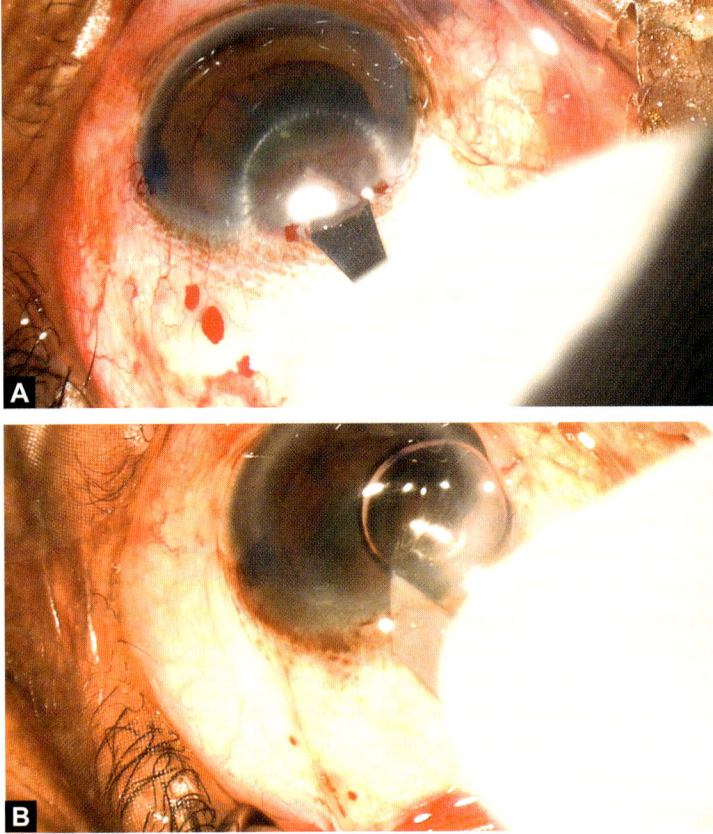

Figs. 3A and B

Results

- Use of blunt instrument is noticed.
- Descemet's membrane can get detached.

Do's
Always use sharp instruments.

Observation (Figs. 4A and B)

Keratome entry is far away from limbus.

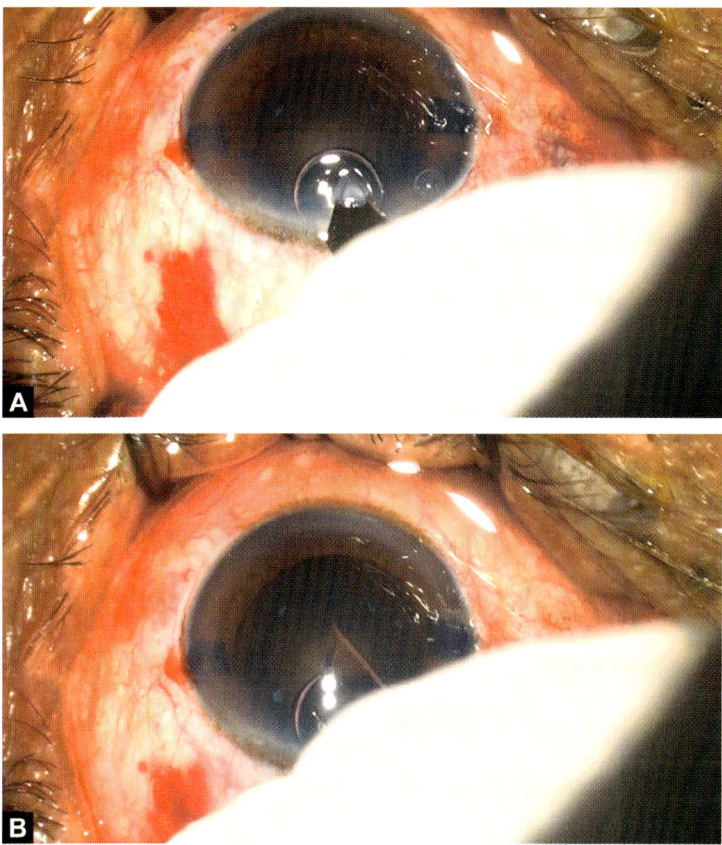

Figs. 4A and B

Result

Phaco surgery can be difficult to perform, mainly capsulorhexis, nucleus management, and irrigation aspiration.

Do's
Keratome entry should be near to limbus for better instrument manipulation.

Observations (Figs. 5A and B)

- Difficulty to pass keratome.
- This situation generally occurs in hypotony.
- Big air bubble is seen which means that anterior chamber is not formed fully with viscoelastics.

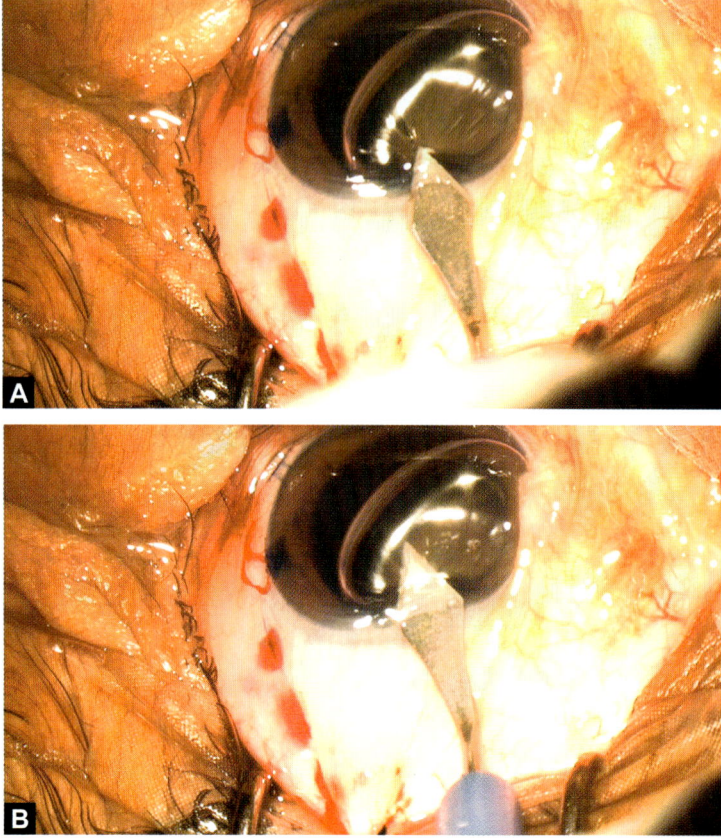

Figs. 5A and B

Results

- Descemet's membrane can get detached.
- More pressure is needed to complete the entry of keratome which can injure anterior capsule.

Do's
Hypotony of eyeball should be converted to normotensive eyeball by filling with viscoelastics.

Observations (Figs. 6A and B)

- Keratome is coming out after completion of incision.
- Corneal touch with keratome tip is noticed.
- Anterior chamber is collapsed.

Incision

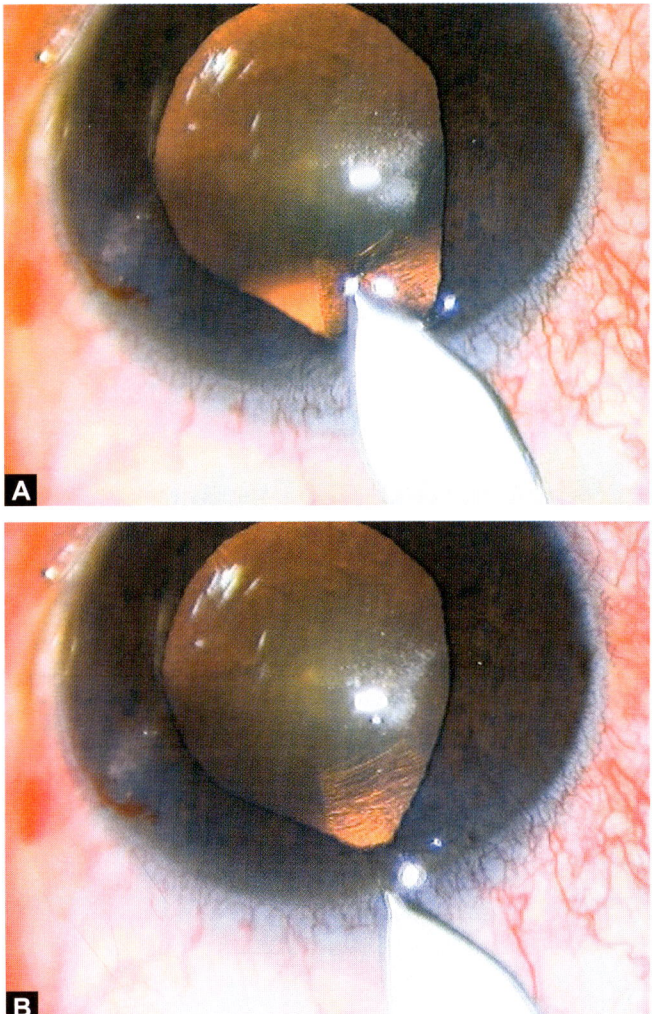

Figs. 6A and B

Result

Injury to cornea, iris or anterior capsule can occur.

Do's
- *This situation happens due to slow movement of keratome while coming out.*
- *Adequate speed is mandatory after completion of incision.*

Observation (Fig. 7)

Length of incision is more in the layers of cornea without anterior chamber entry.

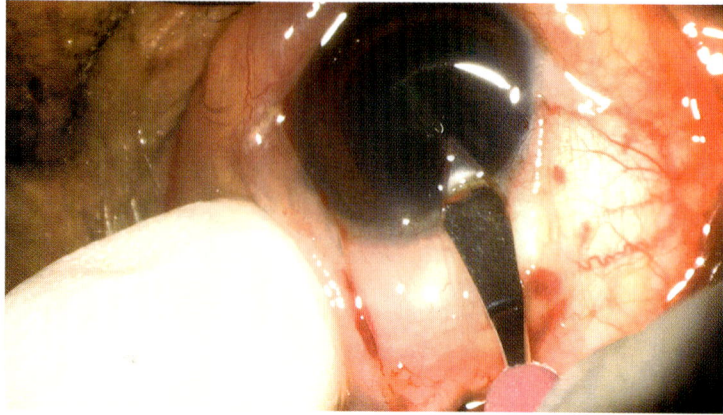

Fig. 7

Result

Long length of incision will interfere with entry and movement of instruments like phaco tip, irrigating/aspirating cannula, intraocular lens (IOL) injector, etc.

> **Do's**
> Length of incision in the layers of cornea should be adequate so that incision should be near square shaped.

Observations (Figs. 8A and B)

- Keratome has been passed fully almost near to 6 o'clock position.
- Direction of keratome is away from center.

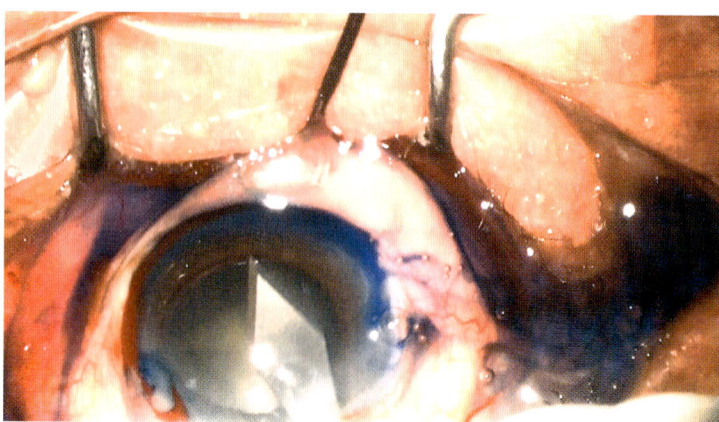

Fig. 8A

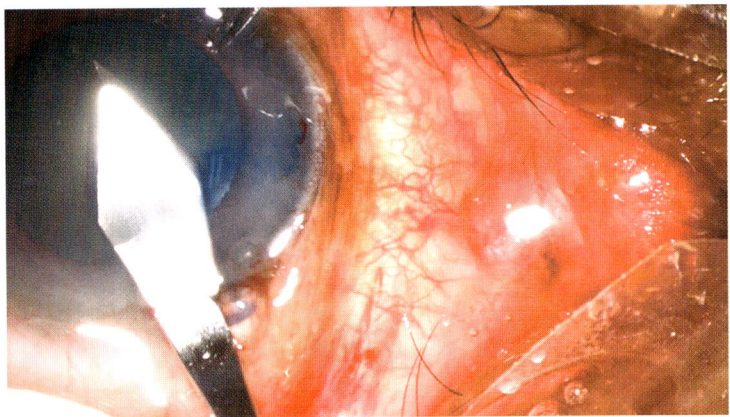

Fig. 8B

Results

- More pressure can cause injury to cornea, iris, and anterior capsule.
- Wrong direction may lead to difficulty to pass phaco tip toward center.

Do's
- Direction of keratome should be towards center.
- Avoid force while passing keratome.
- Such type of force is due to use of blunt instruments, so avoid use of blunt instruments.

Observation (Figs. 9A and B)

Main incision and side port incision is closer to each other.

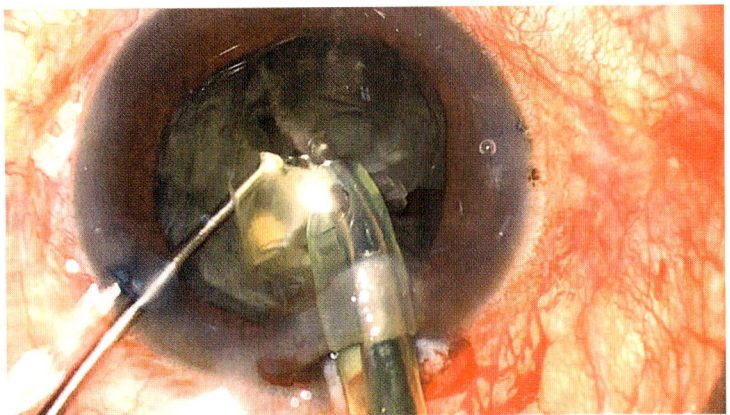

Fig. 9A

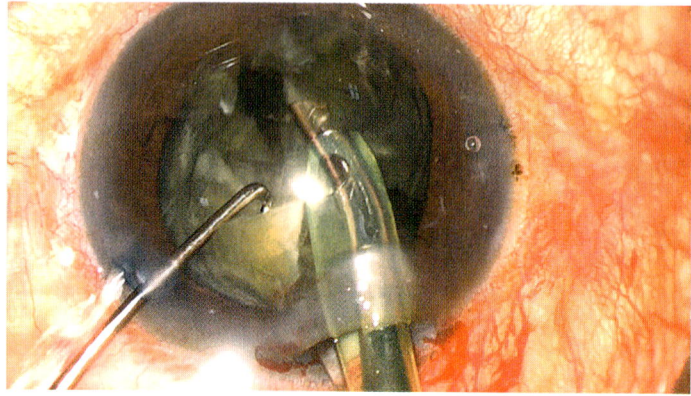

Fig. 9B

Results

- During phaco surgery, leaking of solution occurs through side port.
- Anterior chamber can get collapsed.
- Phaco fluidics can get hampered.

Do's
Distance between main incision and side port incision should be adequate.

CRESCENT

Observations (Fig. 10)

- This is limbal incision.
- Crescent is blunt as folds on cornea seen.

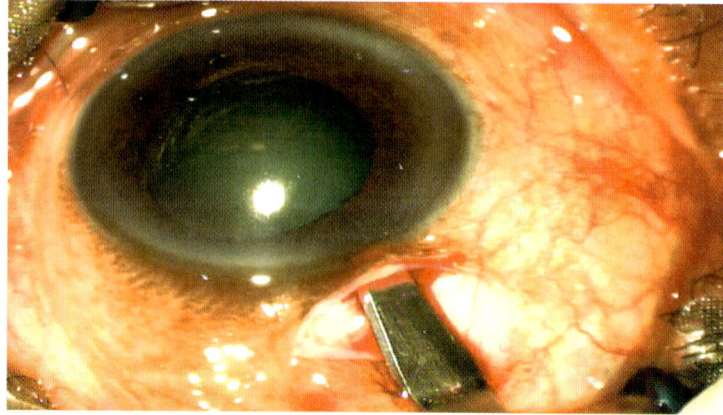

Fig. 10

Result

- Difficulty to do the procedure.

> ***Do's***
> *Crescent should be adequately sharp.*

Observation (Figs. 11A to D)

Crescent is used in tilted fashion during limbal (Figs. 11A and B) and clear corneal incision (Figs. 11C and D).

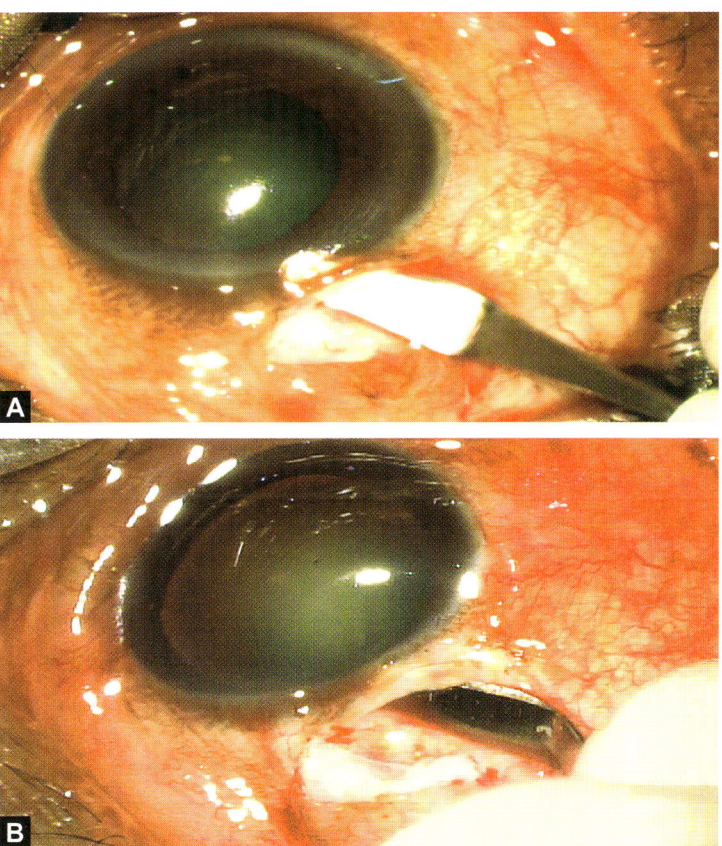

Figs. 11A and B

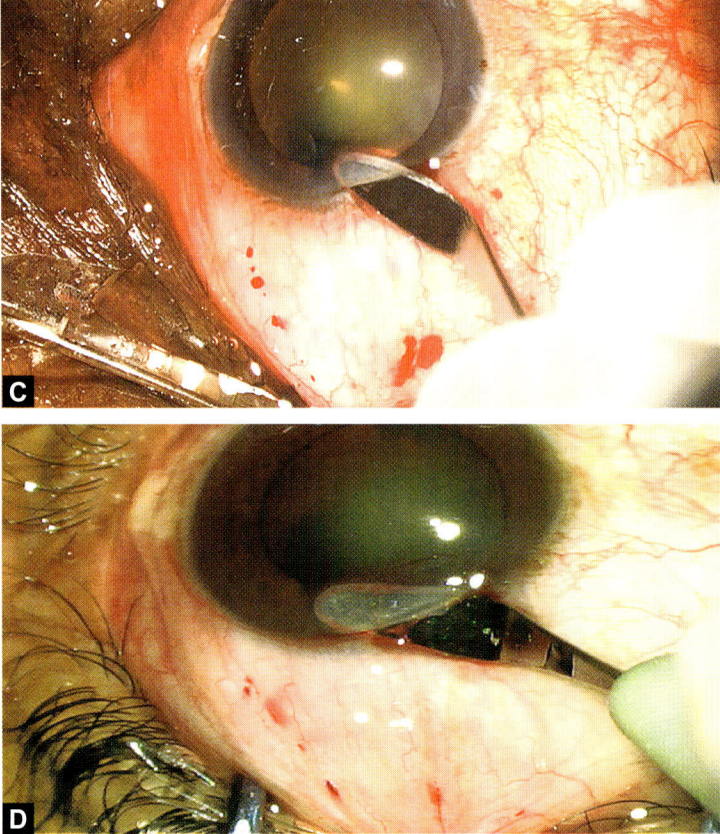

Figs. 11C and D

Results

- Injury to cornea can occur.
- Some time incision can split in vertical fashion.

Do's
Plane of crescent should be parallel to layers of cornea.

SIDE PORT INCISION

Observation (Fig. 12)

Blade is blunt as pressure on cornea is noticed.

Incision

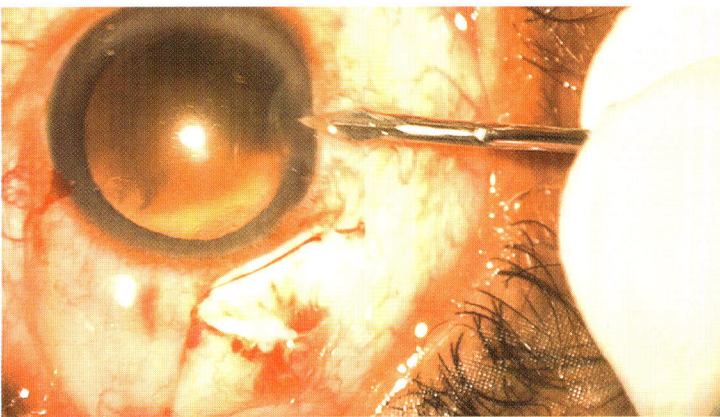

Fig. 12

Result
Difficulty to do incision.

Do's
Instruments should be sharp.

Observation (Fig. 13)
MVR blade is used for right side port incision in tilted fashion.

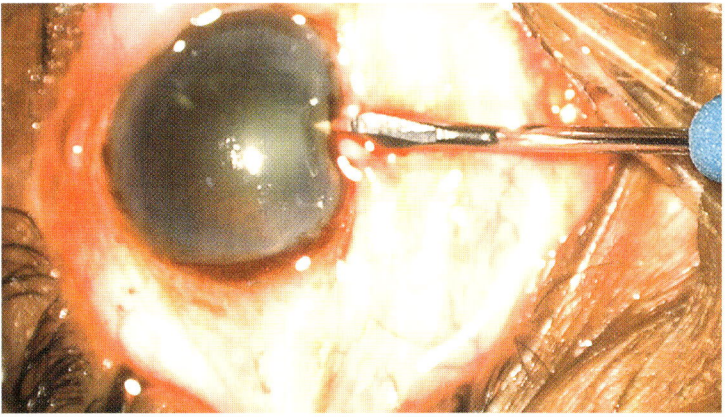

Fig. 13

Result
Injury to cornea can occur.

Do's
MVR blade should be parallel to layers of cornea.

Observation (Figs. 14A and B)

Curved MVR blade is hitting iris.

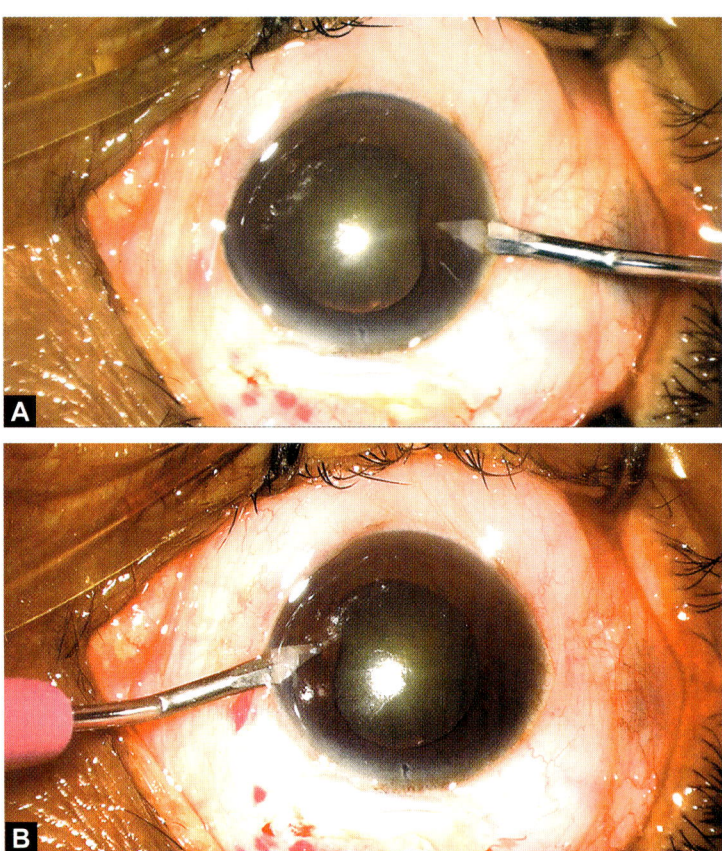

Figs. 14A and B

Results

- Injury to iris can occur in mechanical way or iridodialysis.
- Constriction of pupil can occur which leads to difficulty in further steps.
- Hyphema can occur.

Do's
MVR blade should pass parallel to the iris plane.

CHAPTER 2

Capsulorhexis

INTRODUCTION

Capsulorhexis is one of the most important steps in phaco surgery.

Without normal capsulorhexis, surgeon cannot proceed confidently for phaco surgery.

This is the first step where surgeon actually touches the lens to understand anatomy of the lens (feel of capsulorhexis).

Capsulorhexis can be done by needle, Utrata capsulorhexis forcep, Toshniwal microcapsulorhexis forcep (by Sunayana Surgicals and Segal Optiks, India), and sometimes vannas scissors or micro scissors are needed for this step.

PREPARATION FOR CAPSULORHEXIS

Observation (Fig. 1)

Surgeon is hitting corneal lamellae with cannula.

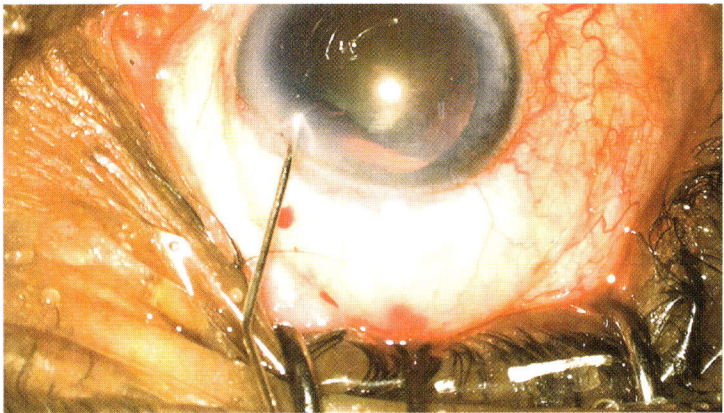

Fig. 1

Result

Descemet's membrane can get detached.

> **Do's**
> - *Cannula should be passed parallel to iris.*
> - *Angulation between cannula and incision site should be perfect.*

Observation (Fig. 2)

Tip of cannula is not visualized.

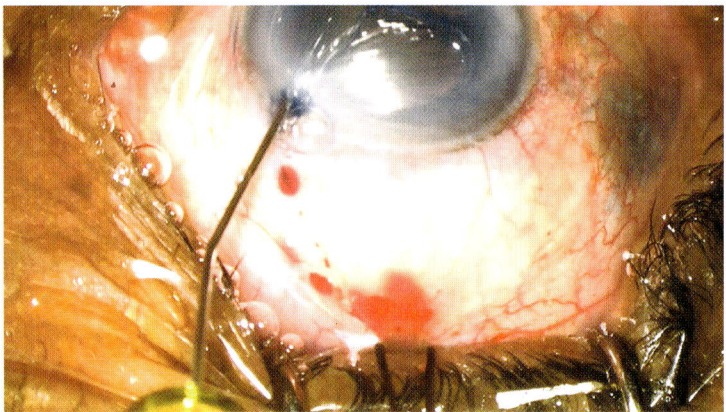

Fig. 2

Result

Descemet's membrane can get detached.

> **Do's**
> *One should always see the distal end of cannula before passing air bubble or trypan blue solution.*

Observations (Figs. 3A and B)

- Stretching of side port incision.
- Folds on cornea seen.

Capsulorhexis

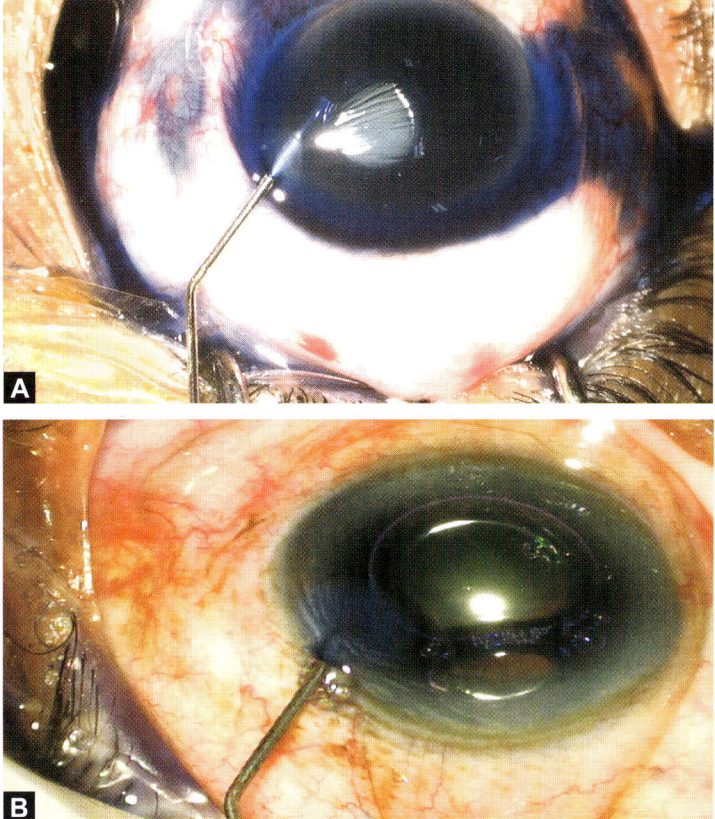

Figs. 3A and B

Result

Injury to cornea can occur.

Do's
Pass cannula through incision at 90° or near 90° to avoid stretching.

Observation (Figs. 4A to C)

Cannula is hitting iris.

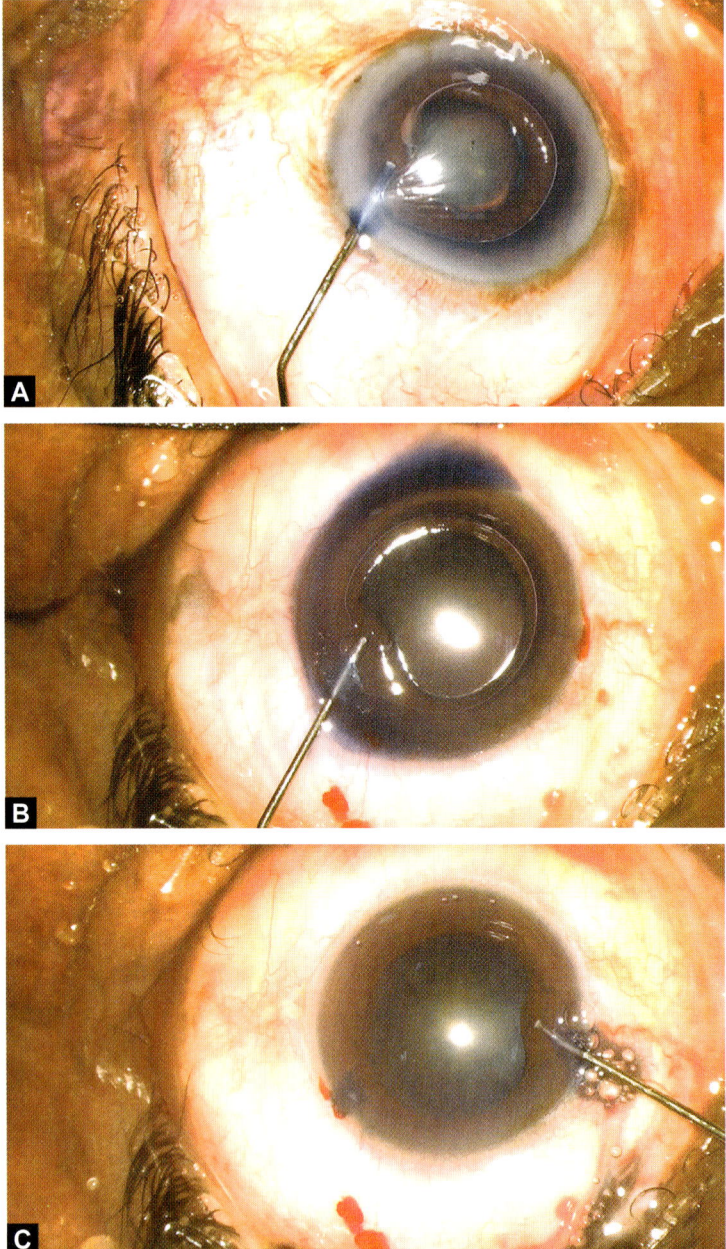

Figs. 4A to C

Results

- Pupil can get constricted.
- Injury to iris can occur.

- Iridodialysis can occur.
- Hyphema can occur.

Do's
Viscoelastics should be put once surgeon enters through side port incision, which settles iris down. After this, put more viscoelastics to form normal anterior chamber.

VISCOELASTICS MIX WITH TRYPAN BLUE

Observations (Fig. 5)

- Anterior chamber is mixed with hyaluron + trypan blue and may be aqueous.
- Bluish discoloration is seen.

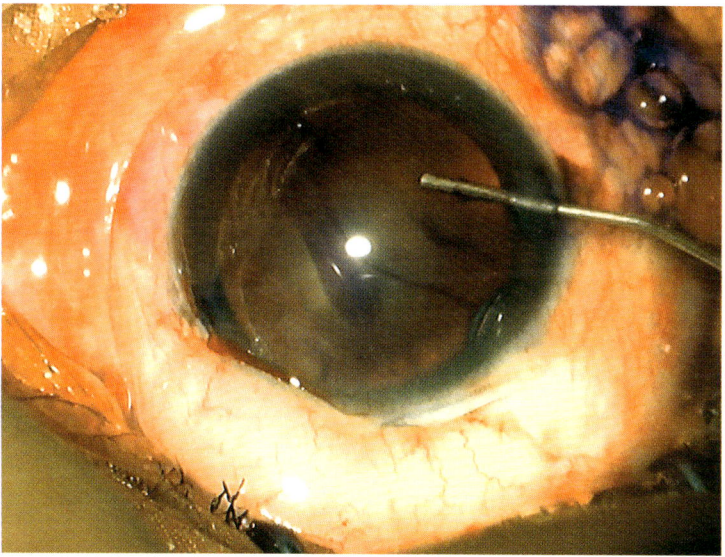

Fig. 5

Result

Visualization during procedure is not good.

Do's
- *Anterior chamber should be transparent.*
- *Putting trypan blue and other viscoelastics is an art.*

CAPSULORHEXIS BY NEEDLE THROUGH SIDE PORT

Observations (Figs. 6A to J)

- Distal end of needle is too long.

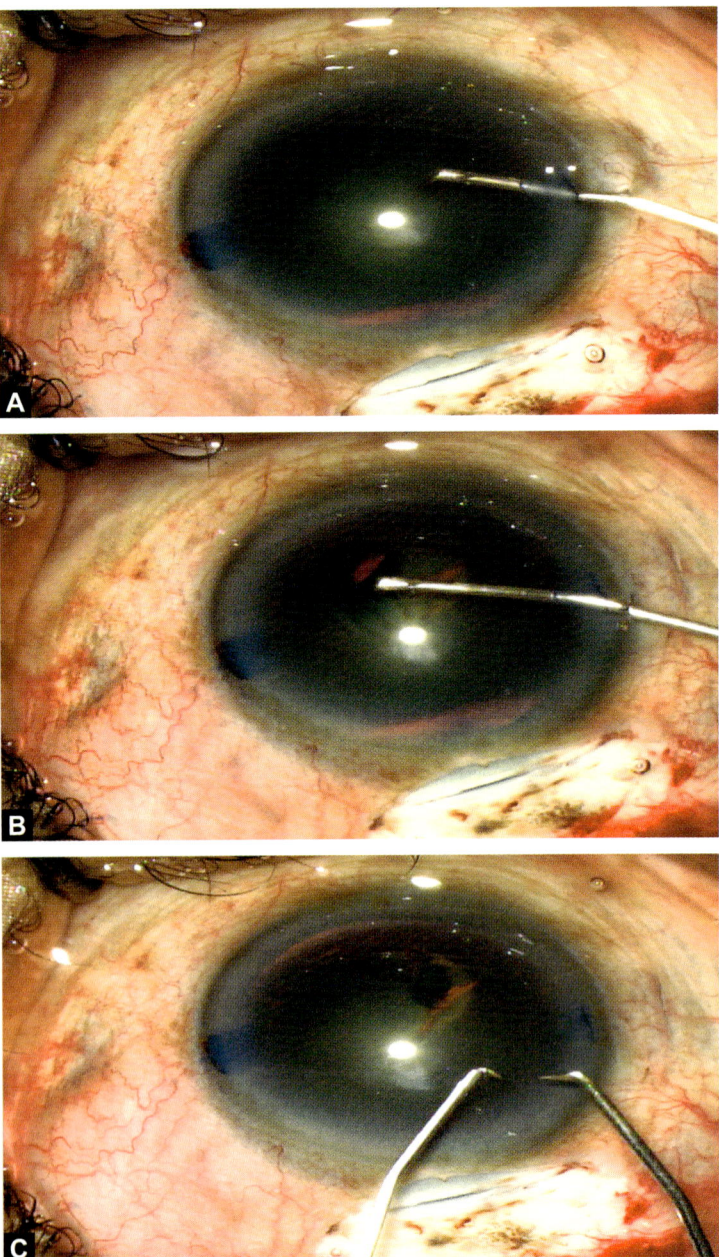

Figs. 6A to C

Capsulorhexis

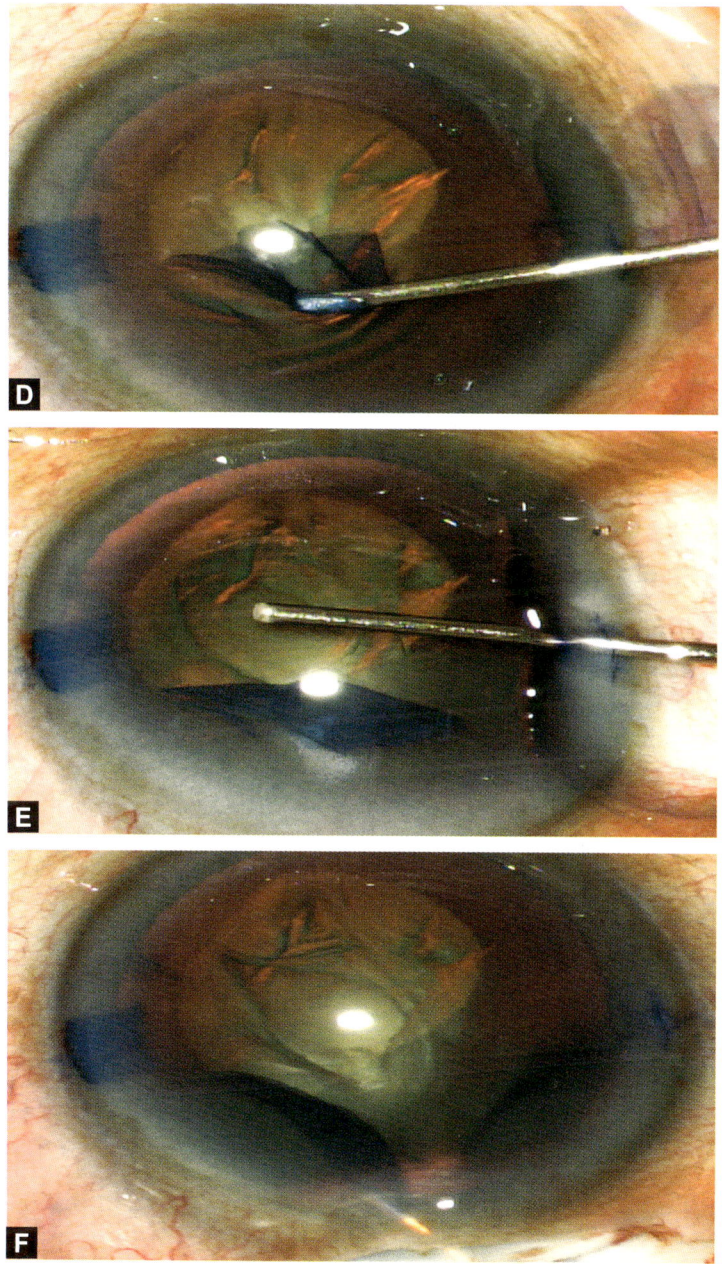

Figs. 6D to F

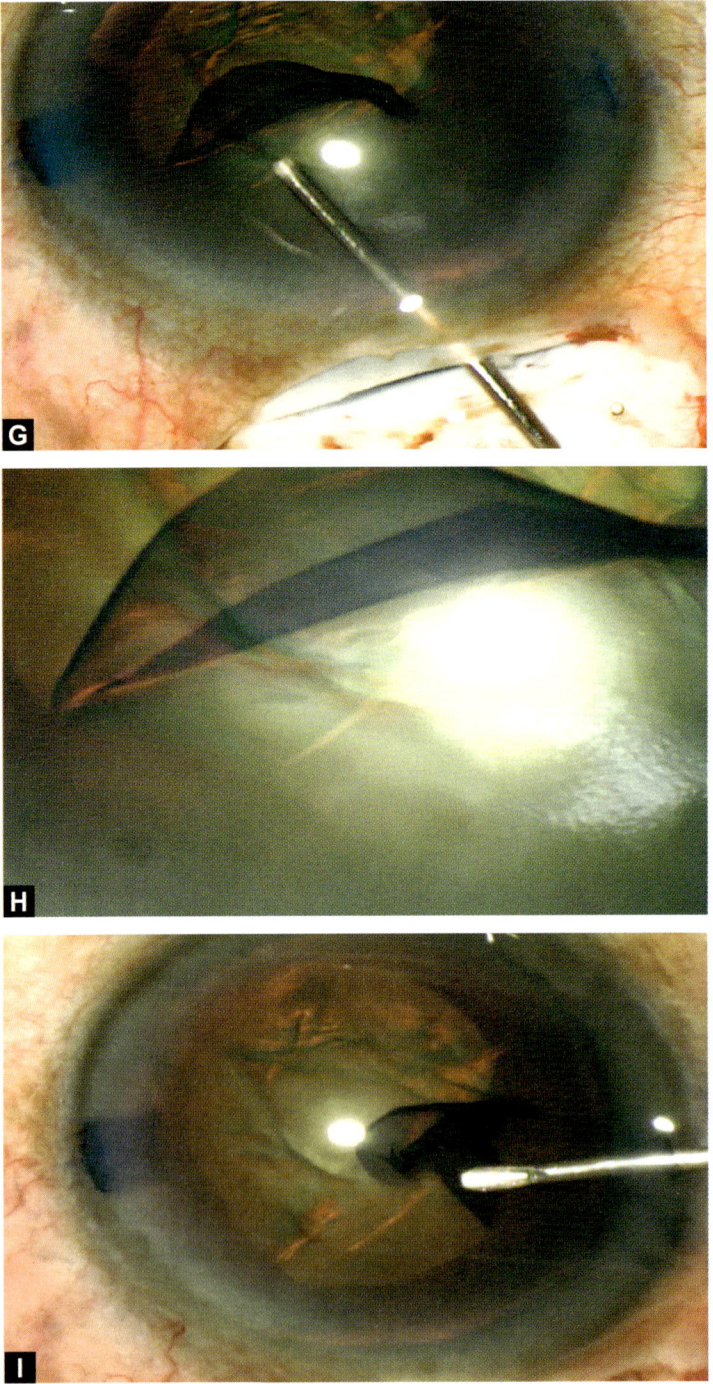

Figs. 6G to I

Capsulorhexis

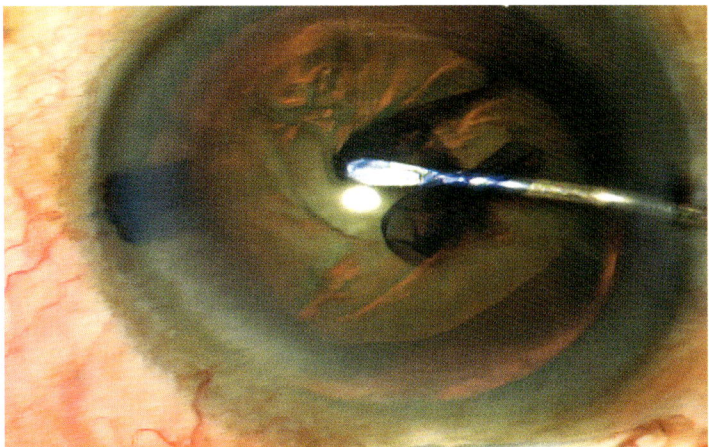

Fig. 6J

- Touching of capsule away from base.
- Capsule is stretched toward main port.
- Putting viscoelastics in a wrong way which results in stretching of capsule.

Results

- Injury to cornea or anterior capsule can occur due to long distal end of needle.
- Capsulorhexis may run away due to stretching of capsule toward main port.

Do's
- Adequate length of needle tip is important for procedure.
- Catching at base of capsule for controlled procedure.
- Putting viscoelastics to relax the capsule is important.
- Adequate speed of procedure is crucial factor for betterment of this step and sometimes speed should be fast or slow (Ref. book Simplified Phacoemulsifition).
- Anterior chamber is very well-maintained throughout procedure due to use of needle.

CAPSULORHEXIS BY UTRATA FORCEP

Observation (Fig. 7)

Capsulorhexis done by forcep through main port.

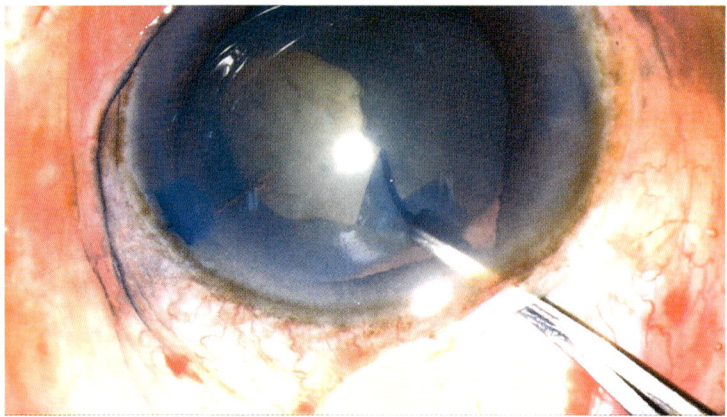

Fig. 7

Result

Anterior chamber can get shallow due to leakage of viscoelastics through main incision and big instrument.

> *Do's*
> - *Capsulorhexis preferably done by needle or microcapsulorhexis forcep.*
> - *One should use heavy viscoelastics like sodium hyaluronate and sodium chondroitin sulfate for this step.*

CAPSULORHEXIS BY NEEDLE AND FORCEP

Observations (Figs. 8A to C)

- Needle passed through edge of main incision to start capsulorhexis.

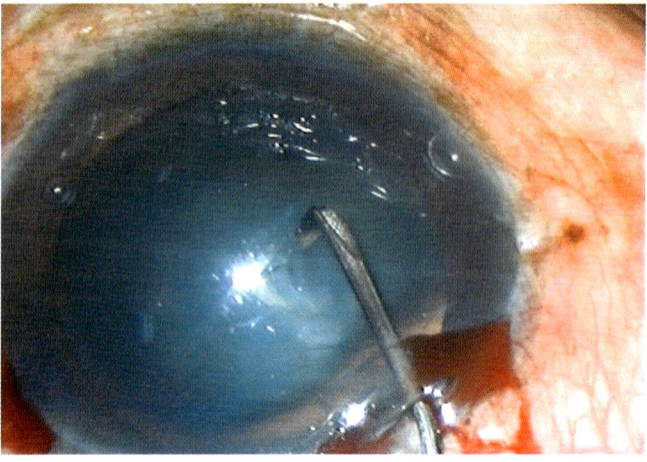

Fig. 8A

Capsulorhexis

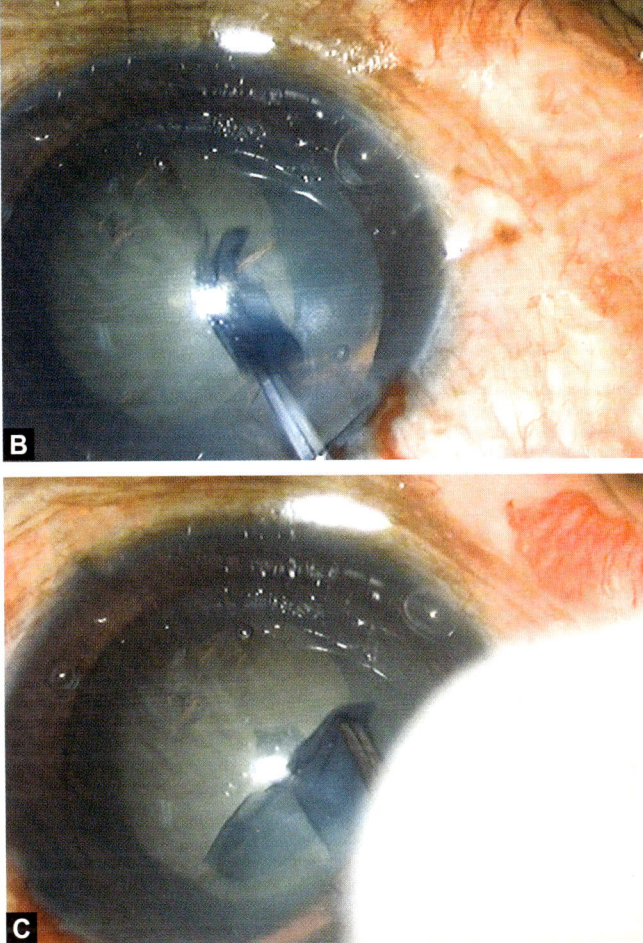

Figs. 8B and C

- Capsulorhexis through main port which is continued by capsulorhexis forcep.
- Hand is seen in the microscopic view.

Results

- Needle movement can get stucked due to entry near edge.
- Capsulorhexis can run away due to nonvisualization and more pressure of forcep.

Do's
- Needle should pass through center of incision.
- Hold the forcep properly.
- Angulation of hand also matters during procedure.

CAPSULORHEXIS BY TOSHNIWAL MICROCAPSULO-RHEXIS FORCEP THROUGH SIDE PORT

Observations (Figs. 9A to F)

- Toshniwal microcapsulorhexis forcep is used for capsulorhexis.
- Catching of capsule away from base is noticed.
- Edge of capsule is not visualized during procedure.
- Folds on capsule are noticed due to wrong way of pulling capsule.

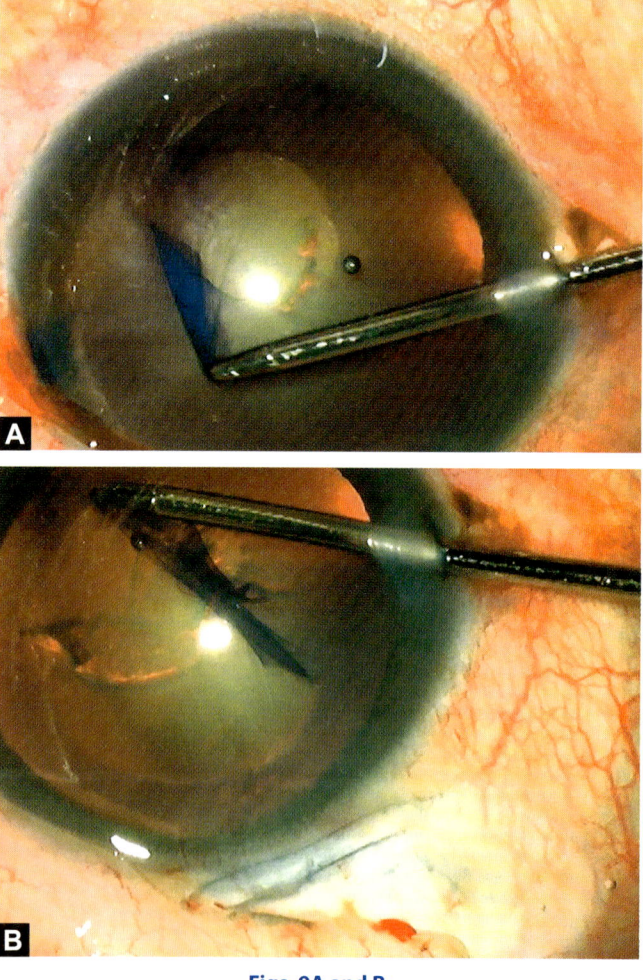

Figs. 9A and B

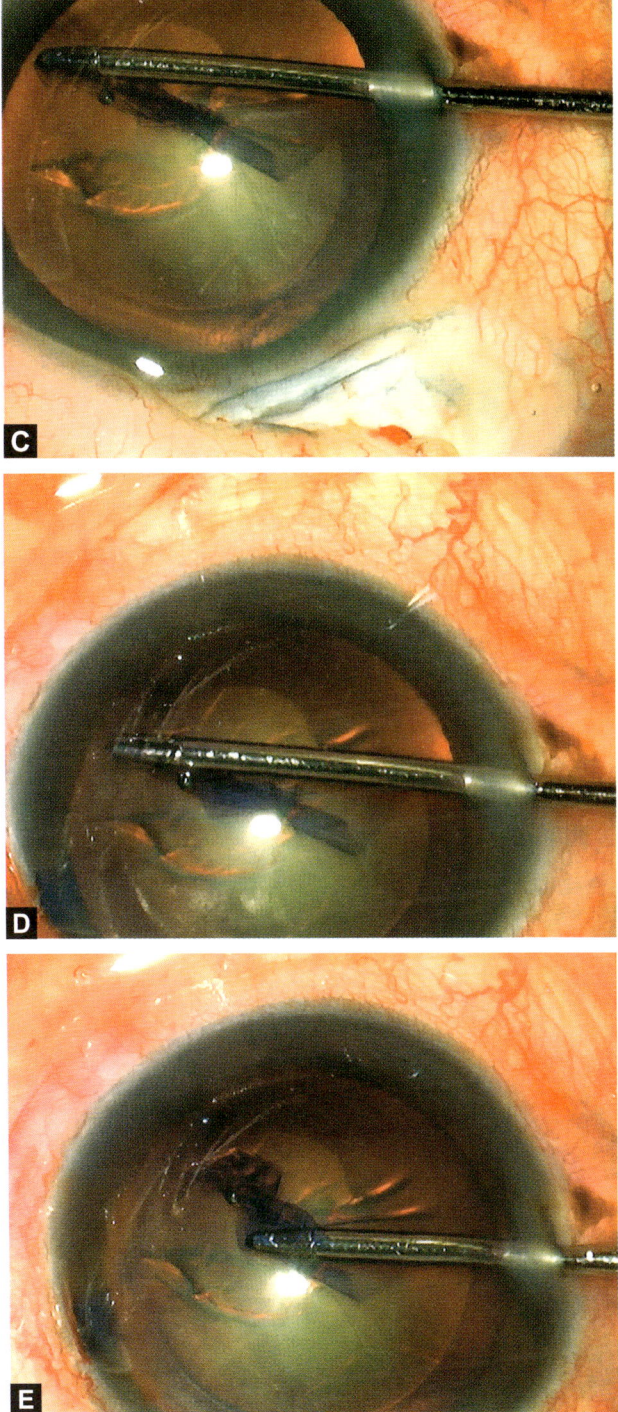

Figs. 9C to E

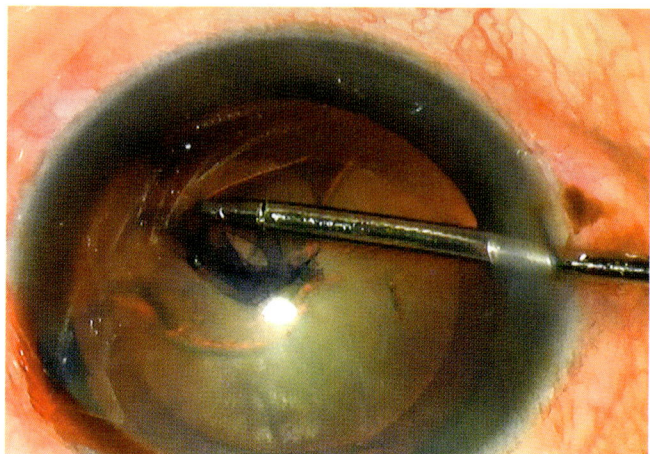

Fig. 9F

Results

Capsulorhexis can run away during procedure due to:
- Nonvisualization
- Wrong pull on capsule.

Do's
- *Capsulorhexis procedure is done under strict visualization.*
- *Catching the base of capsulorhexis for controlled procedure.*
- *Such a type of instrument is having advantage of needle as well as forceps.*

CAPSULORHEXIS THROUGH SIDE PORT – DIFFERENT SITUATIONS

Observation (Fig. 10)

Needle is passing beneath the capsule.

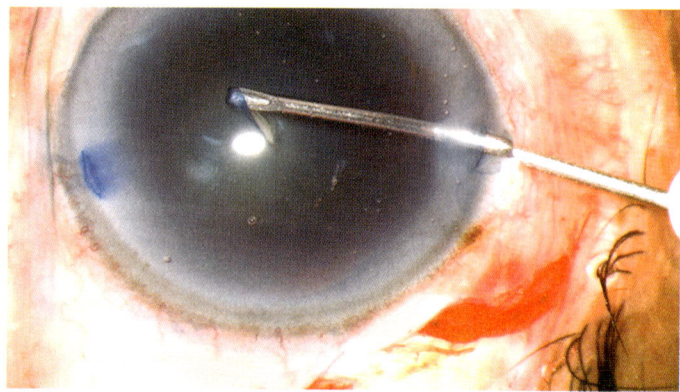

Fig. 10

Result

Capsule can get torn in abnormal way.

> **Do's**
> Touch the capsule anteriorly during start of capsulorhexis.

Observation (Figs. 11A and B)

Folds on anterior capsule seen due to touch of blunt needle and micro-capsulorhexis forcep.

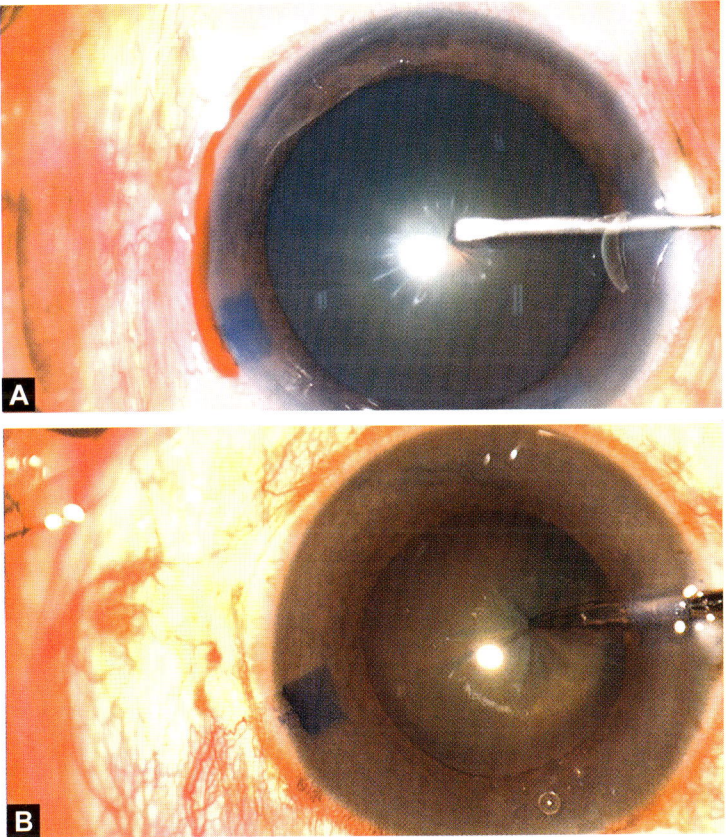

Figs. 11A and B

Results

- Stretching on capsule can occur.
- Opening of capsule is difficult.

> **Do's**
> - Sharp instrument or needle is mandatory to open the capsule.
> - Open the capsule by sharp needle and continue with microcapsulorhexis forcep.

Observation (Fig. 12)

Edge of capsule is not seen.

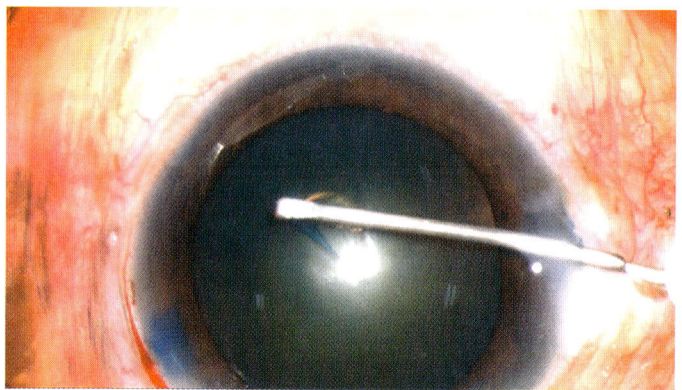

Fig. 12

Result

Capsule open in abnormal direction.

> **Do's**
> Needle should touch edge of capsule under visualization.

Observation (Fig. 13)

Viscoelastics is coming out through side port.

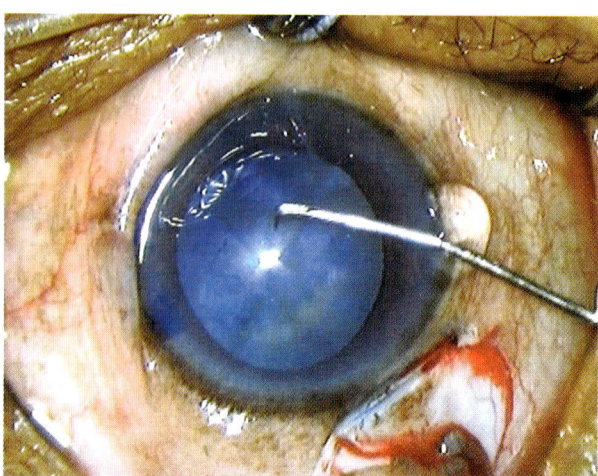

Fig. 13

Result

Anterior chamber can get shallow.

> *Do's*
> - *This situation can occur due to:*
>   - *More pressure of needle at incision site.*
>   - *Putting more viscoelastics in anterior chamber than needed.*
>   - *Anatomically pre-existing shallow anterior chamber.*
> - *Avoid pressure by needle at start of procedure.*
> - *Adequate viscoelastics should be put in anterior chamber before start of capsulorhexis.*

Observation (Fig. 14)

Needle is passed in oblique way.

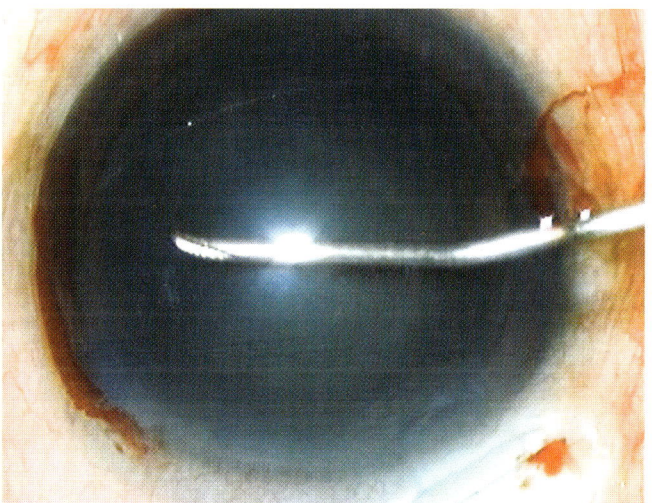

Fig. 14

Results

- Anterior capsule can open peripherally.
- Capsule can cut in abnormal way.

> *Do's*
> - *Pass needle horizontally with direction of tip toward surgeon.*
> - *Needle will open capsule in vertical fashion.*
> - *Continue procedure in oblique direction of needle.*

Observations (Figs. 15A and B)

- More pressure by needle during capsulorhexis as folds on cornea seen.
- Needle is placed in wrong direction and well away from edge of capsule.

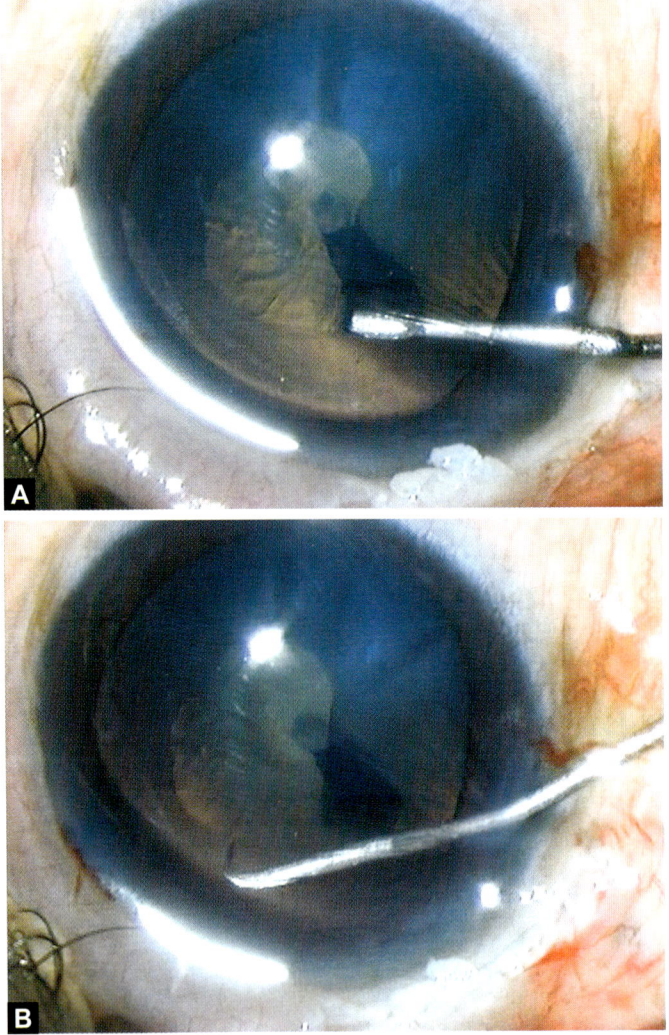

Figs. 15A and B

Results

- Visualization is hampered due to pressure.
- Needle can damage cornea or anterior capsule.

Do's
- *Avoid pressure during capsulorhexis.*
- *Needle should work near the edge of capsule.*

Observation (Figs. 16A and B)

Needle touching the capsule at center.

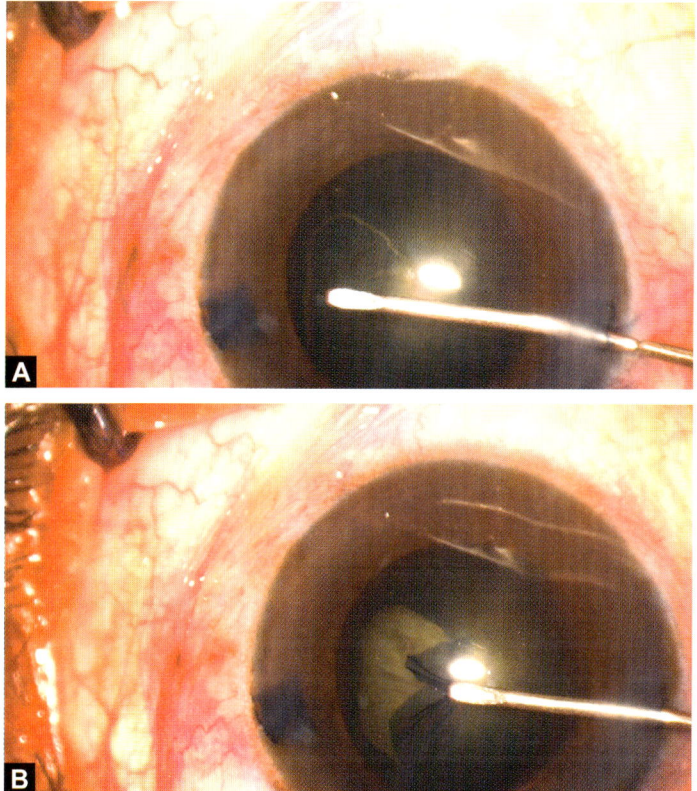

Figs. 16A and B

Results

- Peeling of anterior capsule from two sides.
- Capsulorhexis can run away.

Do's
Continue the capsulorhexis from one edge of opened capsule.

Observations (Figs. 17A to D)

- Started the capsulorhexis from periphery.
- Microcapsulorhexis forcep is passing vertically through side port incision in acute angle.
- Surgeon using more force to enter, so that hitting the capsule in the periphery near the incision.

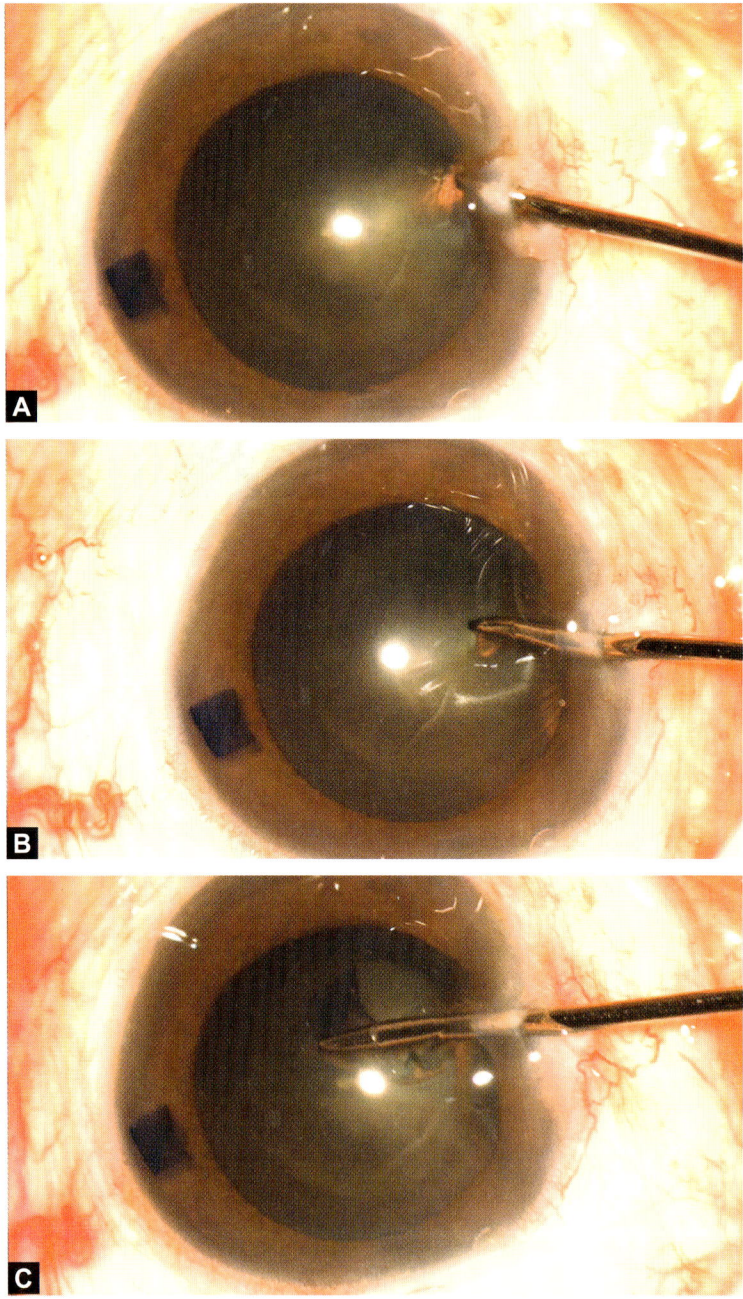

Figs. 17A to C

Capsulorhexis

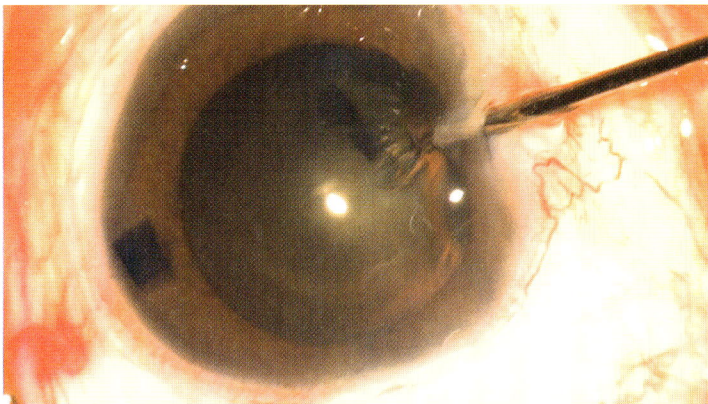

Fig. 17D

Results

- Restricted movement of forcep due to long incision.
- Vertical stretching of side port incision is seen.
- Due to folds on cornea, visualization is hampered.

Do's
- *Side port incision should be of adequate length and width.*
- *Microcapsulorhexis forcep should pass horizontally.*
- *Start the capsulorhexis from center.*

CAPSULORHEXIS THROUGH MAIN PORT – DIFFERENT SITUATIONS

Observation (Fig. 18)

Difficulty to pass needle through main port.

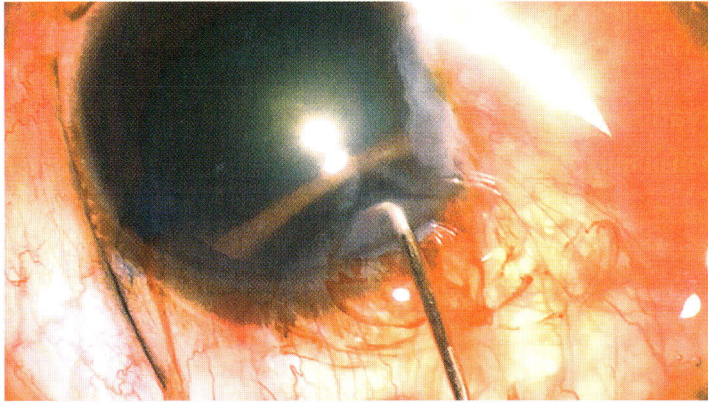

Fig. 18

Result

Can damage Descemet's membrane.

> *Do's*
> *Needle should pass through center of incision.*

Observations (Fig. 19)

- Needle passes through main port.
- Visco is coming out through main port.

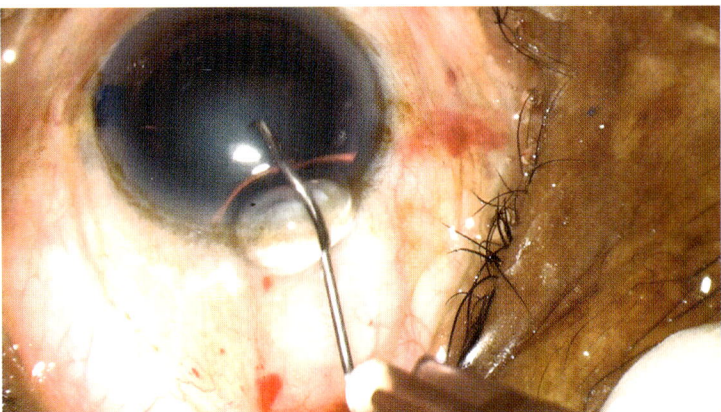

Fig. 19

Result

Anterior chamber can get shallow.

> *Do's*
> *Generally capsulorhexis should be done by needle through side port as main port is big in length.*

Observation (Fig. 20)

Reflection of microscope light is in the view during procedure.

Capsulorhexis 37

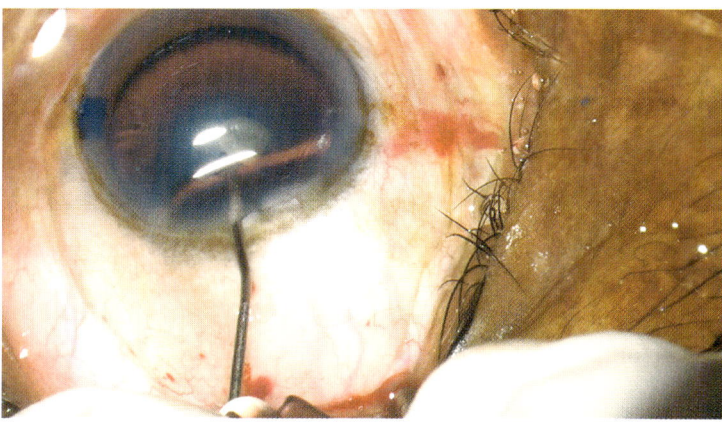

Fig. 20

Result

Capsulorhexis is difficult.

Do's
Tilting of head position to avoid light reflection in the view.

Observation (Fig. 21)

Vertical stretching of wound by needle.

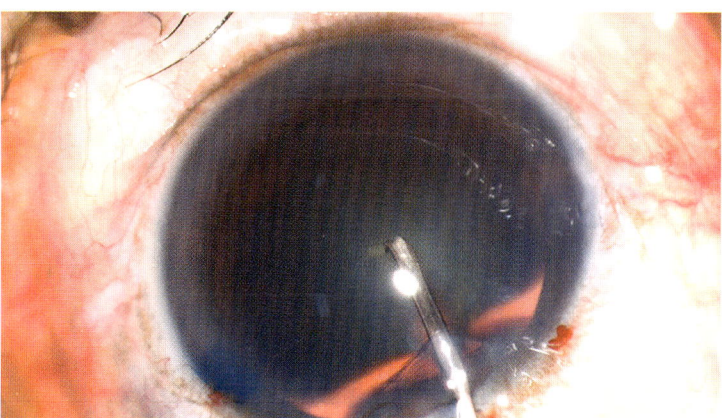

Fig. 21

Result

- Injury to cornea can occur.
- Anterior chamber can get shallow.

Do's

• Pass needle horizontally, then work vertically to start capsulorhexis and pass through center.

Observations (Fig. 22)

- This is a very common finding where capsular flap near main incision and needle in action.
- Acute angulation of needle is noticed.
- Corneal folds are seen.

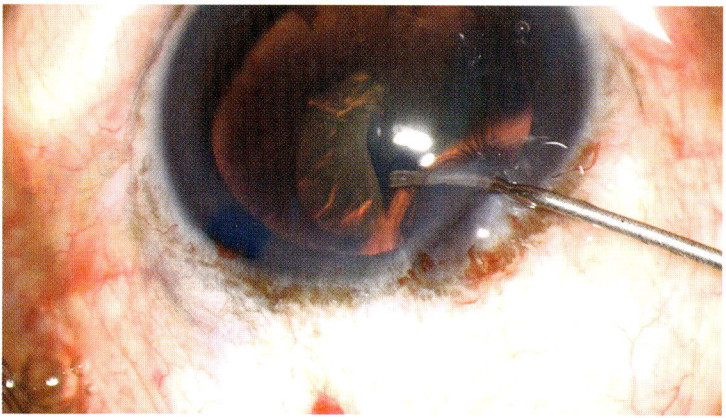

Fig. 22

Result

Capsulorhexis can run away.

Do's

At this point, needle can be used through side port to complete capsulorhexis.

Observation (Fig. 23)

Visco cannula is placed over the flap.

Capsulorhexis

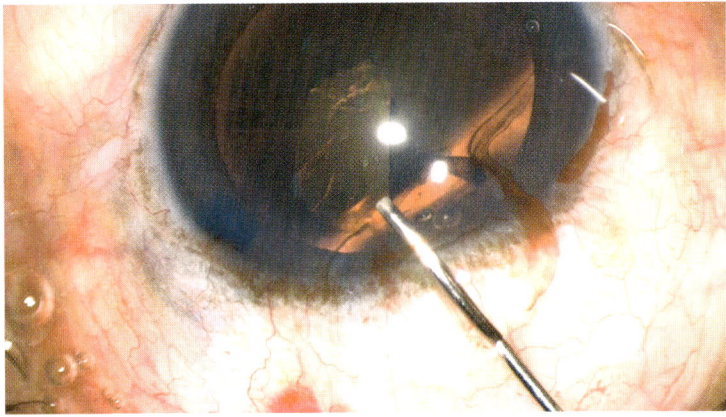

Fig. 23

Result

Capsulorhexis can run away.

Do's
Put the visco in such a way that anterior capsule flap should get settle and relax to complete capsulorhexis.

Observation (Fig. 24)

Capsule is stretched toward main incision.

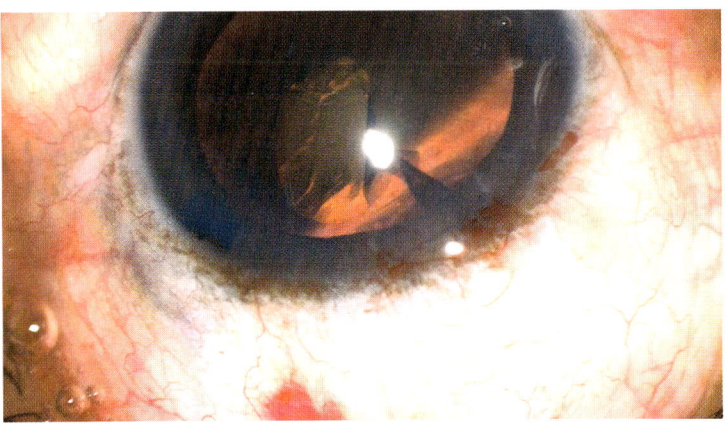

Fig. 24

Result

Capsulorhexis can run away.

Do's
- *This situation happened due to passing of visco through main port in wrong way.*
- *It is an art to put visco through main port to settle or reposition the capsule.*

Observation (Fig. 25)

Iris is catched by forcep.

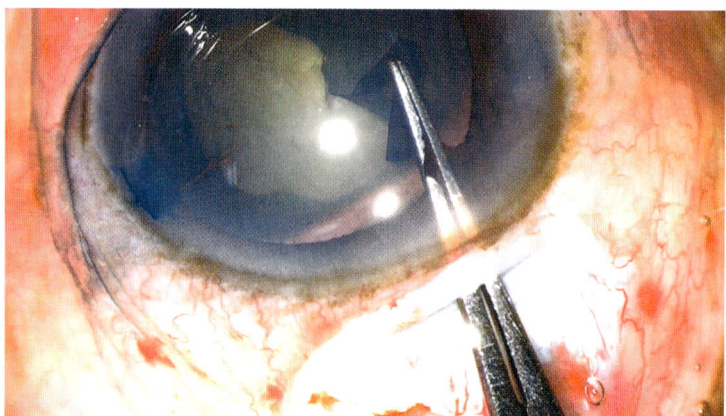

Fig. 25

Result

Injury to iris or iridodialysis can occur.

Do's
Settle the iris by putting visco to form anterior chamber and continue the procedure.

Observation (Fig. 26)

Both edges of capsule have been pulled.

Capsulorhexis

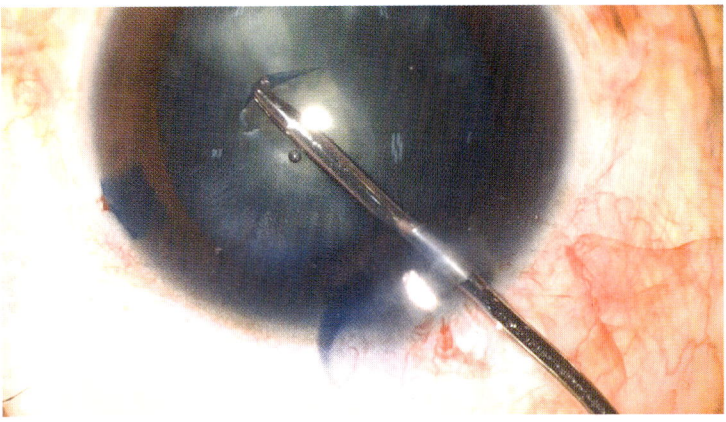

Fig. 26

Result

Capsulorhexis can run away.

Do's
Start the capsulorhexis by catching one edge of torned capsule.

CAPSULORHEXIS IN ONE CASE

Observations (Figs. 27A to F)

- 26 G needle passed vertically from side port.
- Vertical placement of the needle may touch the capsule at a wrong position.

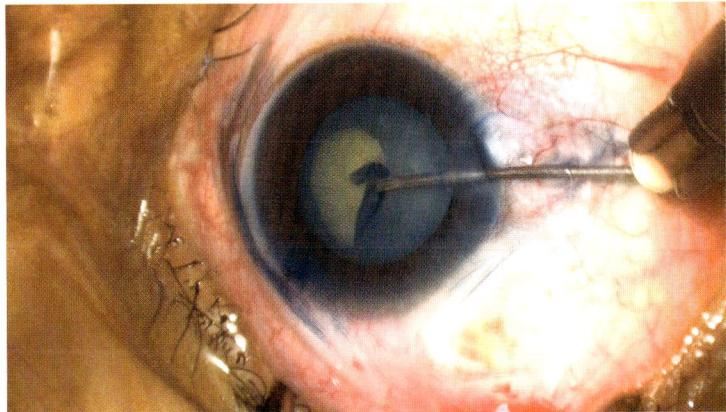

Fig. 27A

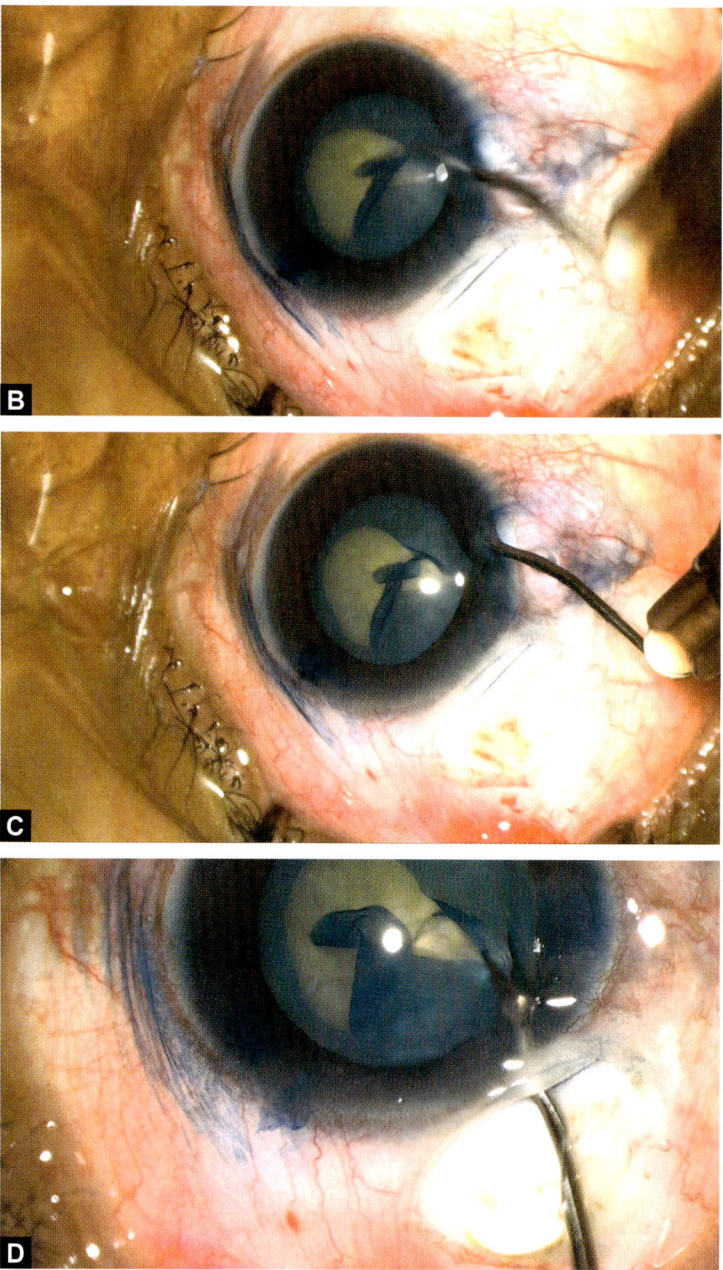

Figs. 27B to D

Capsulorhexis

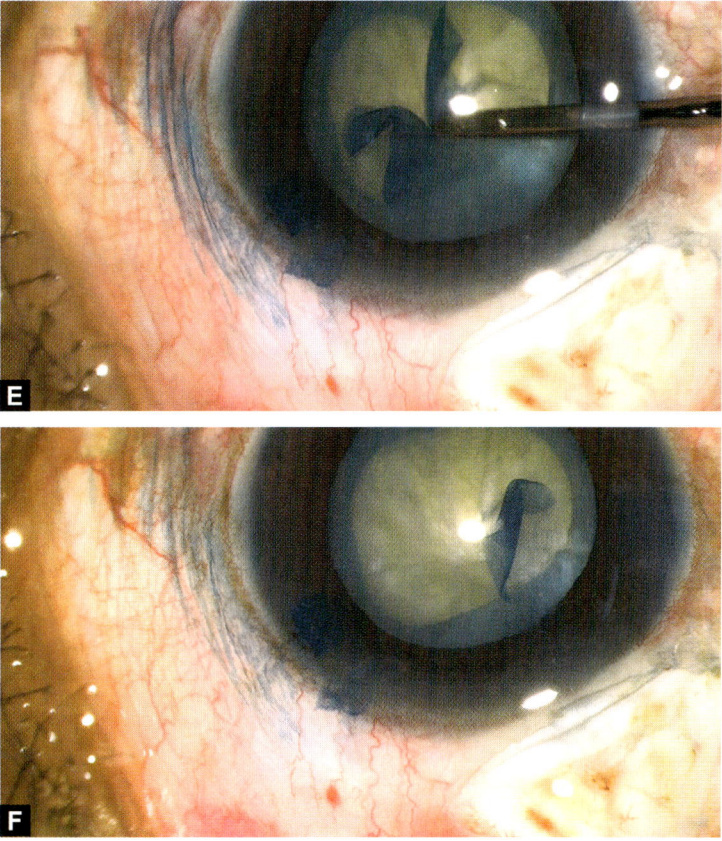

Figs. 27E and F

Result

Capsulorhexis can run away.

> **Do's**
> - Capsulorhexis can be done with vertical placement of needle but one has to be very careful to avoid such situation.
> - Oblique placement of the needle is many times helpful for controlled capsulorhexis.
> - Help of microcapsulorhexis forcep and micro scissor has been taken to complete the capsulorhexis.

CHAPTER 3

Hydroprocedures

INTRODUCTION

- Hydroprocedure is an important step to mobilize the lens before phaco procedure.
- Hydroprocedure can be hydrodelineation, hydrodelamination, and hydrodissection.

HYDRODISSECTION

Observations (Figs. 1A and B)

- Hydrodissection cannula passed from edge of incision.
- Procedure started near main incision area.
- More pressure is noticed at incision site.

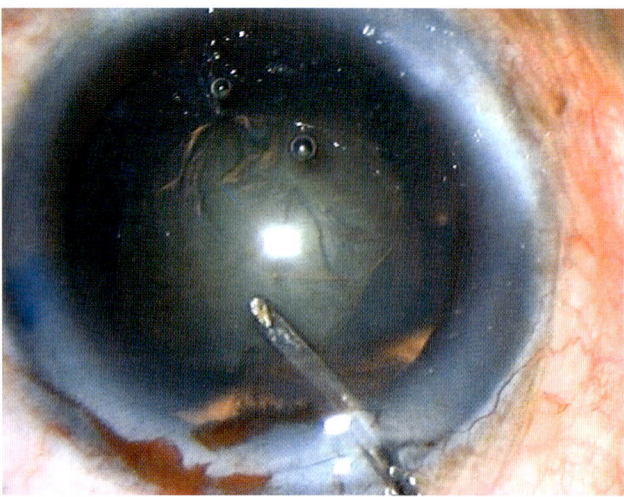

Fig. 1A

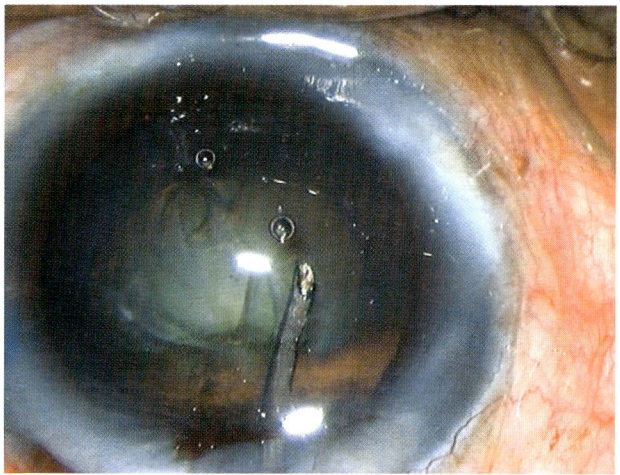

Fig. 1B

Result

- Anterior chamber can get shallow
- Visualization is hampered.

Do's
- *Pass cannula through center of incision.*
- *Procedure should start beneath anterior capsule, away from incision means 3'o clock or 9'o clock for 12'o clock incision site.*
- *Avoid pressure of cannula at incision site for better visualization.*

Observations (Figs. 2A and B)

- Pressure on nucleus is noticed as a mark of cannula over epinucleus (Fig. 2A).
- Incision stretched vertically (Fig. 2B).

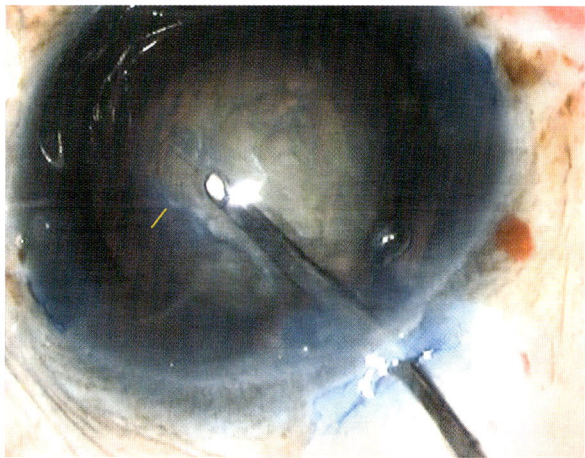

Fig. 2A

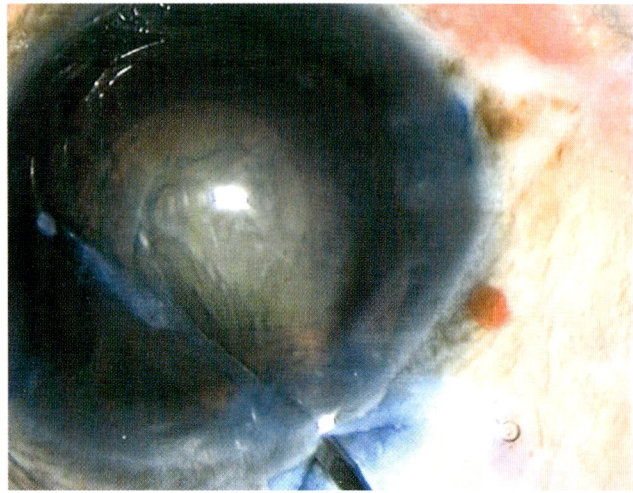

Fig. 2B

Results

- Anterior chamber can get shallow.
- Pressure on lens can weaken zonules.

Do's
Cannula should pass parallel to iris plane.

Observation (Figs. 3A and B)

Distal end of cannula is not seen.

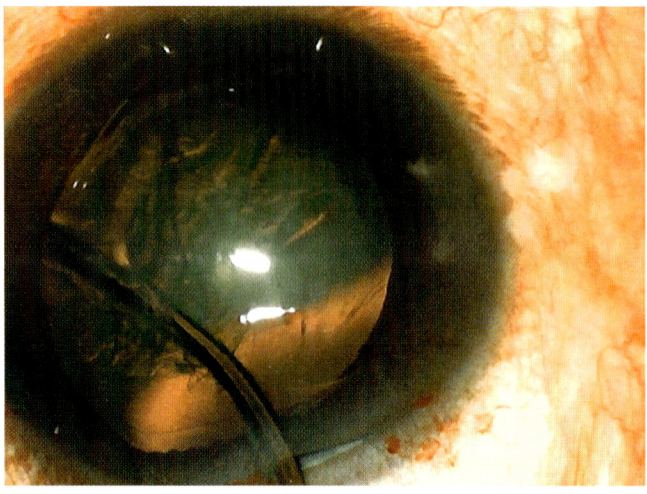

Fig. 3A

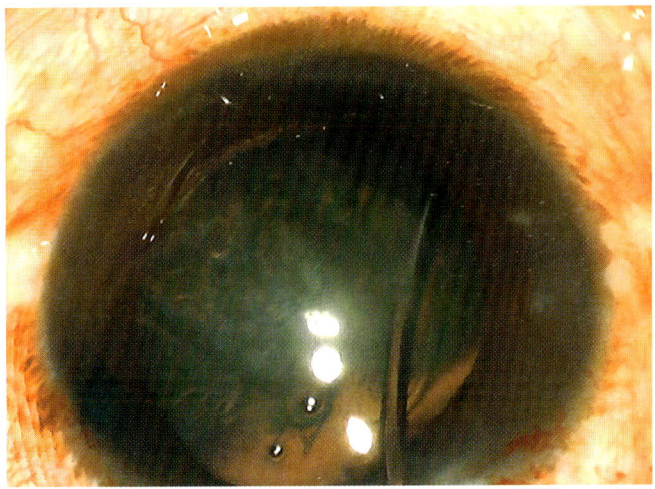

Fig. 3B

Results

- Hydroprocedure is blind and difficult.
- Constriction of pupil can occur.

Do's
Hydrodissection cannula should be visible during procedure.

Observations (Figs. 4A to E)

- Hydrodissection done by cannula through main incision at acute angle.
- Hydrodissection done partially.

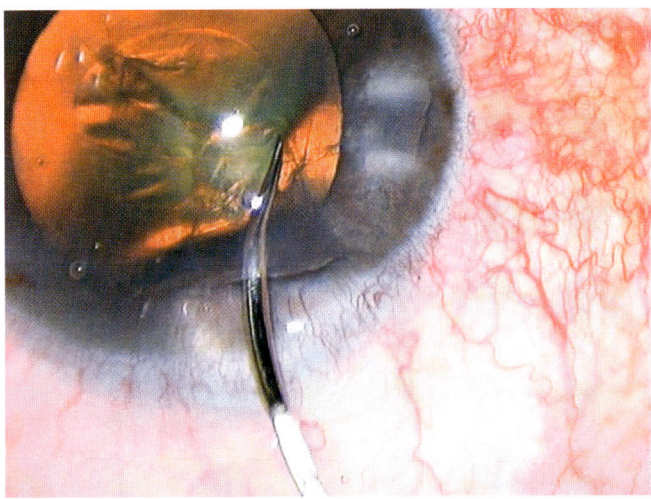

Fig. 4A

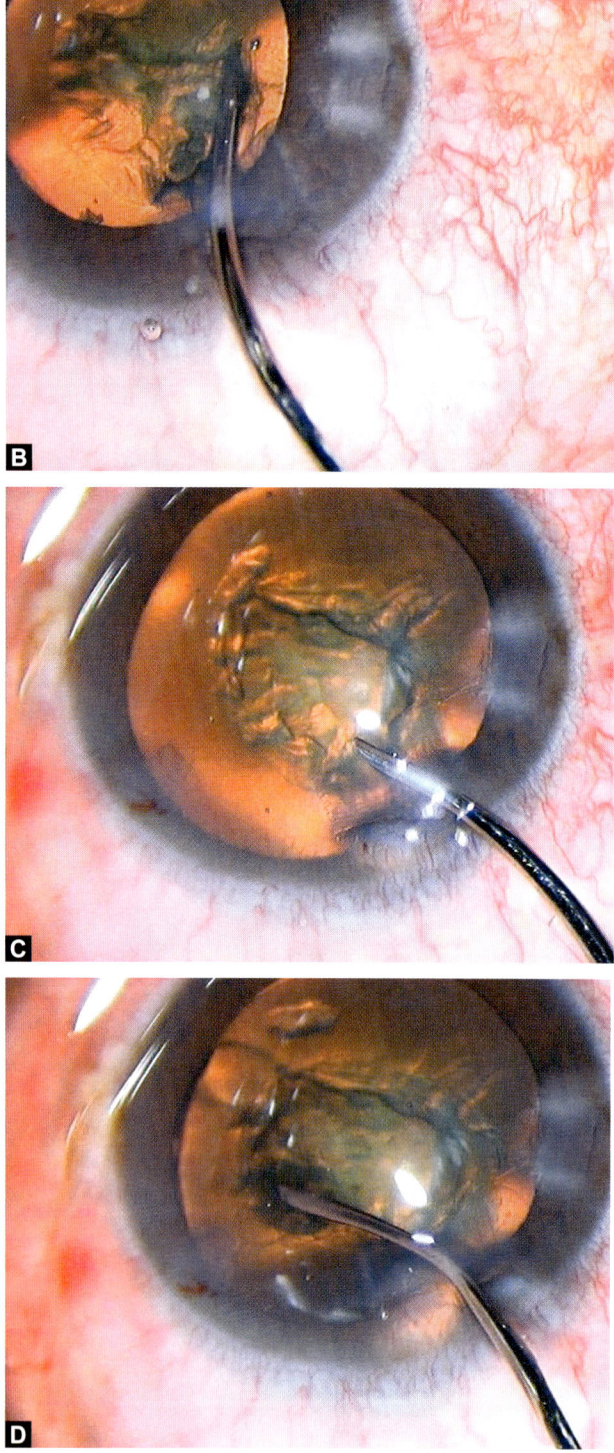

Figs. 4B to D

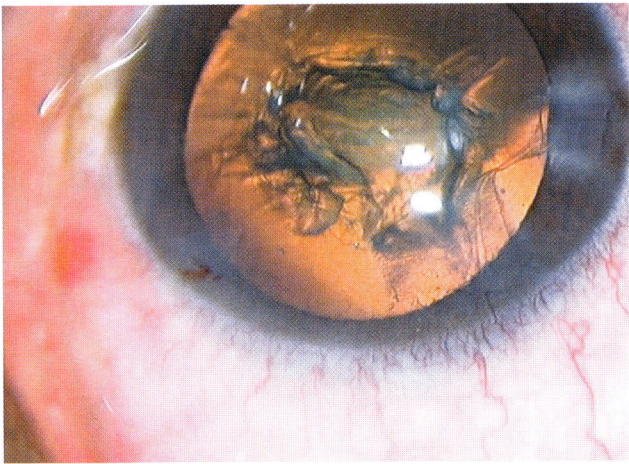

Fig. 4E

Results

- Due to acute angle, procedure is difficult.
- Anterior chamber can get shallow.
- Partial hydrodissection does not serve the purpose of procedure.

Do's
- Start hydrodissection away from main incision.
- Water should pass properly beneath anterior capsule.

HYDRODELINEATION

Observation (Fig. 5)

During hydrodelineation procedure, cannula is seen near to center of nucleus.

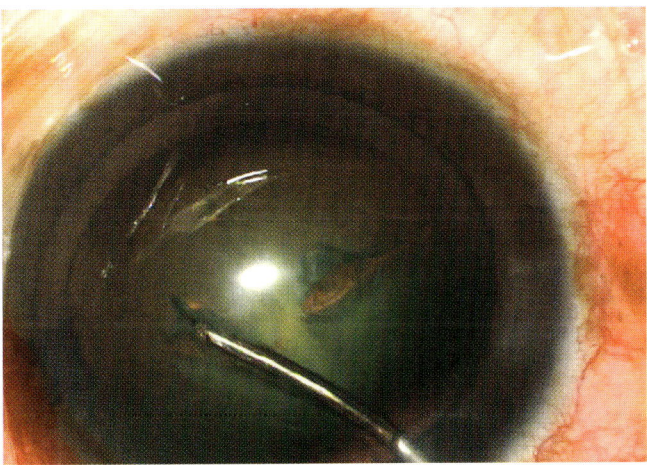

Fig. 5

Result

Golden ring noticed which means hydrodelineation has started.

> **Do's**
> Hydrodelineation should be done by passing cannula in substance and at the edge of nucleus.

Observation (Figs. 6A and B)

Anterior chamber is getting shallow during hydroprocedures.

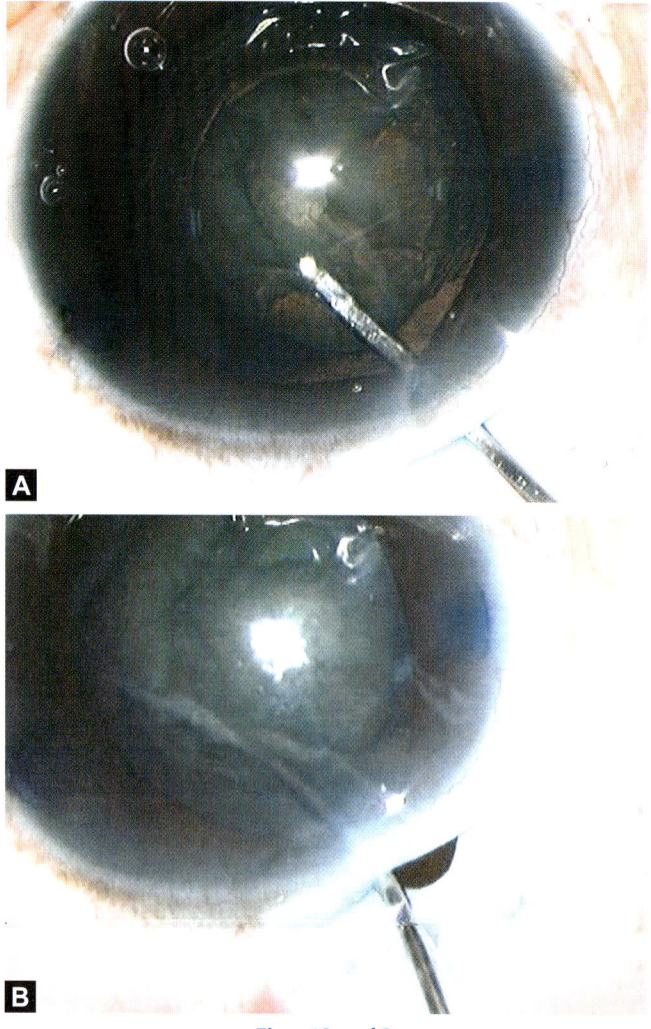

Figs. 6A and B

Result

Iris prolapse can occur.

> **Do's**
> During hydroprocedures, decompression of the lens by tapping over it is very important to avoid such situation.

CHAPTER 4

Trench

INTRODUCTION

- Trench is the first step for stop and chop or divide and conquer technique in nucleus management.
- Phaco tip is generally in bevel up position in this step.
- Adequate energy according to density of nucleus is needed.
- Length and depth of trench depend on size and hardness of nucleus.

Observations (Fig. 1)

- Difficulty in entry of phaco tip before start of trench.
- Eccentric placement of the phaco tip.
- Phaco tip is in bevel up position.

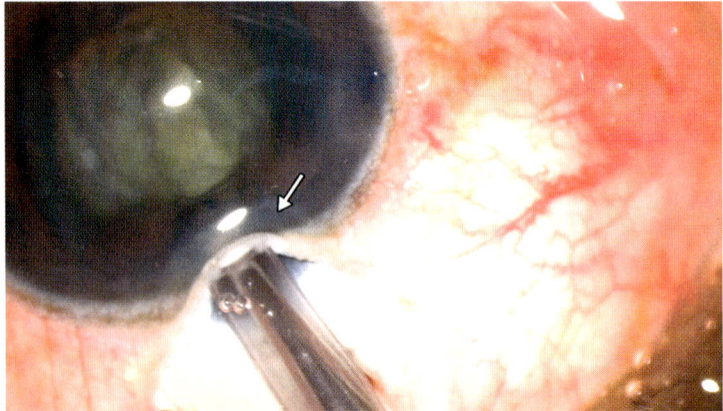

Fig. 1

Result

Descemet's membrane can get detached.

Do's
- Phaco tip should pass three-dimensional (3D) center of incision.
- Angulation of the phaco tip should be parallel or near parallel to iris plane.
- Phaco tip should enter in bevel down or bevel side way in straight tip.

Observations (Figs. 2A to C)
- Phaco tip is stucked at incision.
- Phaco tip touches the iris.
- Exposed part of phaco tip is more without sleeve; it means that sleeve is tucked at incision site.
- Shallowing of anterior chamber is due to no irrigation of fluid.

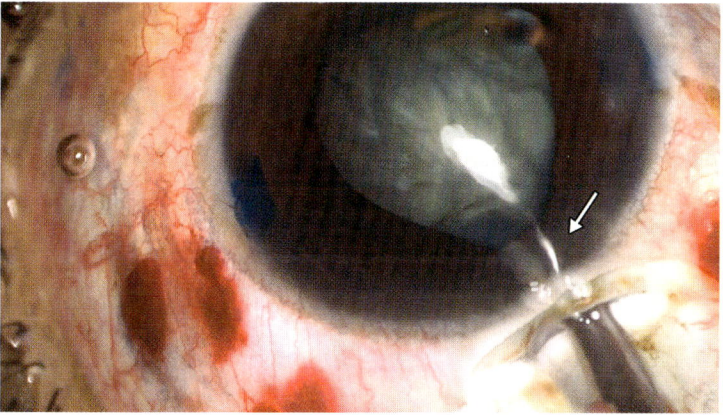

Fig. 2A

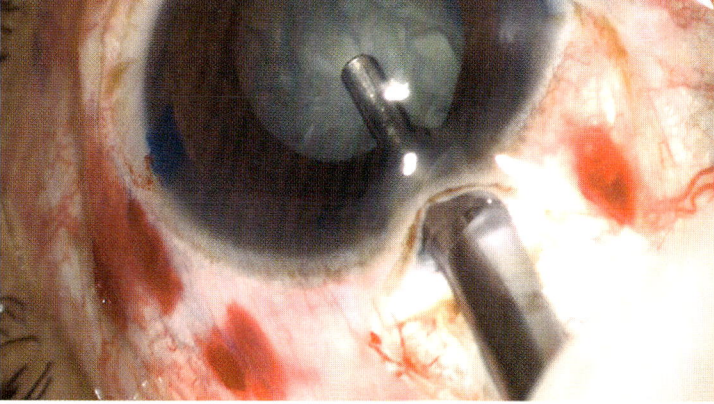

Fig. 2B

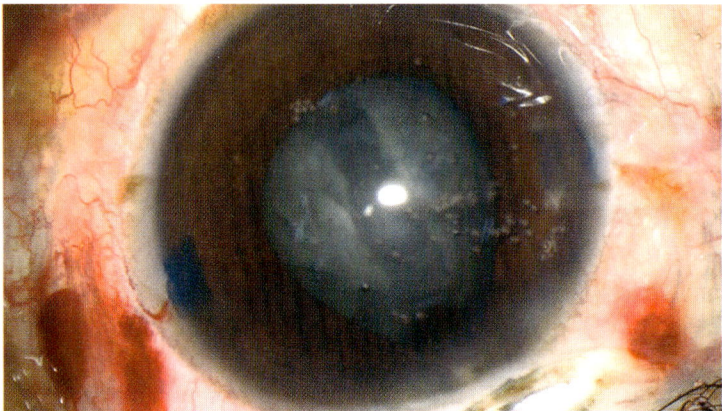

Fig. 2C

Results
- Mechanical injury to cornea and iris can occur.
- Cornea or iris can get burned.

Do's
- *This situation can occur due to:*
  - *Pre-existing shallow anterior chamber.*
  - *Deep plane of incision.*
- *Entry of phaco tip through the incision should be smooth, with adequate speed, and 3D center of incision.*
- *Phaco probe should pass parallel to iris plane and sometimes quick movement is necessary.*
- *Angulation of introducing phaco tip at incision site is very important.*

Observation (Fig. 3)

Iris is stucked during trench.

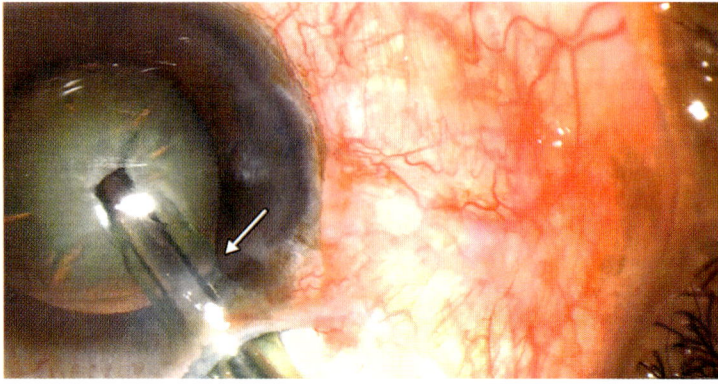

Fig. 3

Results

- Rubbing of the phaco probe can cause iris injury and constriction of pupil.
- Uneven anterior chamber can transmit the energy to cornea.

Do's
- *Phaco probe should pass through normal filled anterior chamber.*
- *Phaco probe should not pass slowly to avoid this situation.*

Observations (Figs. 4A to D)

- Sleeve is stucked at incision site.
- More exposed part of phaco tip is seen.

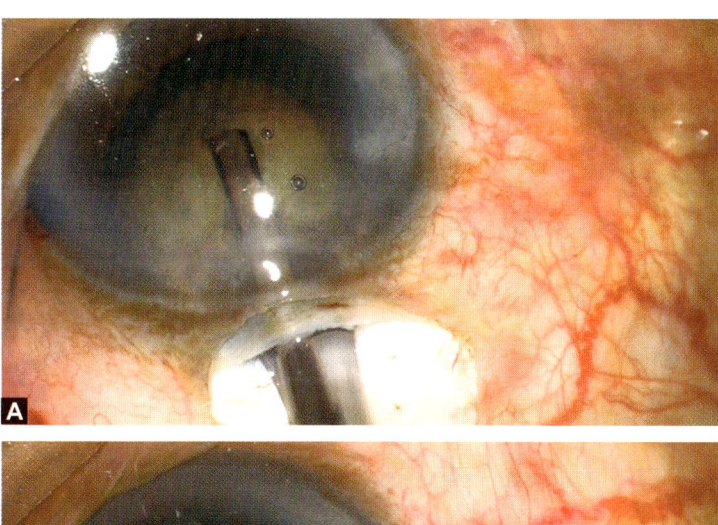
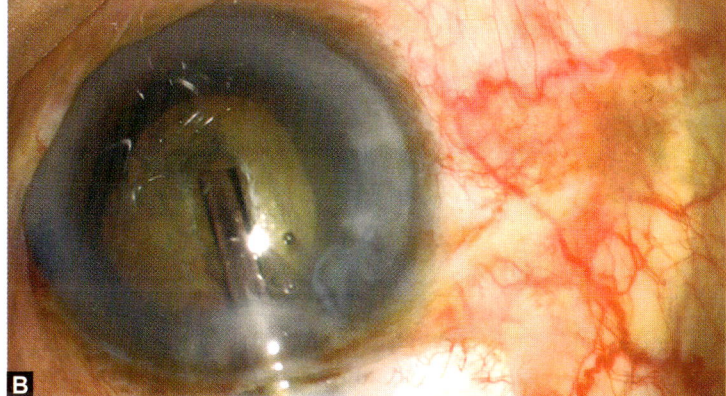

Figs. 4A and B

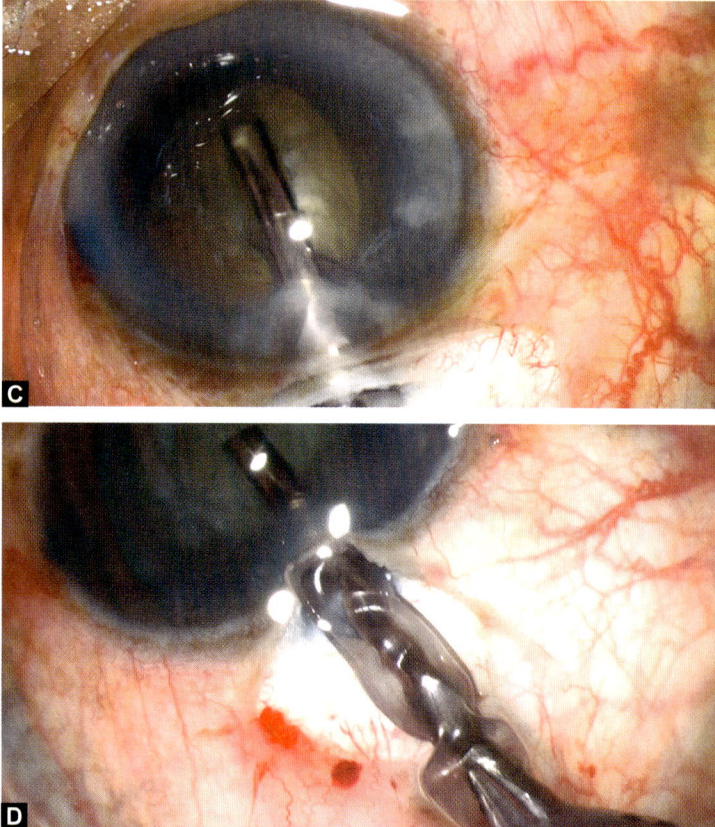

Figs. 4C and D

Result

Corneal burn can occur due to more exposed part of phaco tip and collapsed anterior chamber.

Do's
Confirm the proper entry of phaco tip with sleeve before start of trench.

Observations (Fig. 5)

- Air bubble is seen during trench.
- Air bubbles are due to more heat and friction between water current and viscoelastics.
- Sometimes air bubbles are passed through irrigation line of tubing.

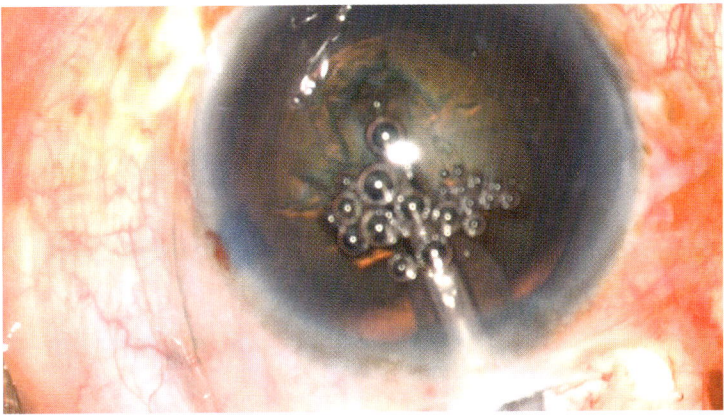

Fig. 5

Result

Visualization of the trench is hampered which can lead to difficulty in this step.

> **Do's**
> - Removal of air bubble can be done by phaco tip in irrigation/aspiration mode or with viscoelastic.
> - Trench should be done after removal of air bubble only for proper visualization of procedure to avoid complications.

Observations (Fig. 6)

- Irrigating fluid seen like wave.
- Surgeon is doing trench superficially.

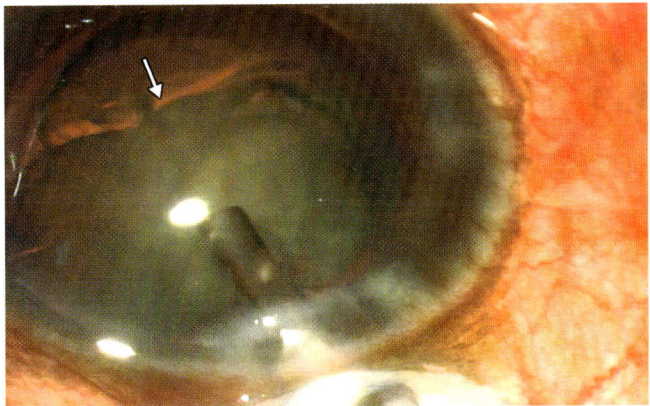

Fig. 6

Result

Corneal burn can occur.

Do's
Trench should start by touching the nucleus.

Observation (Fig. 7)

Sudden entry with more energy in the nucleus material will disturb it and look like shower.

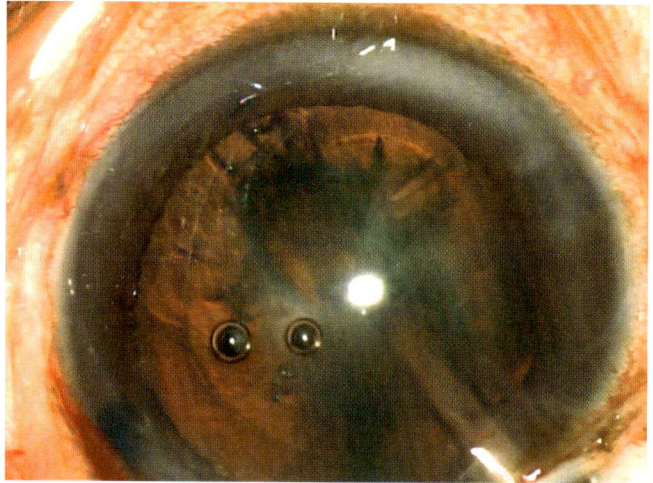

Fig. 7

Result

Visualization is hampered.

Do's
Trench should be done layer by layer with adequate energy.

Observations (Fig. 8)

- Trench started too periphery near incision.
- Wound leakage can occur.

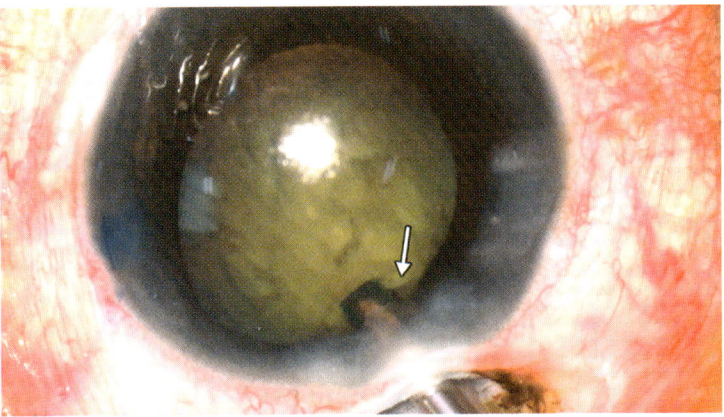

Fig. 8

Result

Injury to cornea or iris can occur.

Do's

Trench should start little away from periphery and according to the size and hardness of nucleus.

Observations (Fig. 9)

- Trench is done with bevel down position.
- In this position, instead of trench hold occurs.

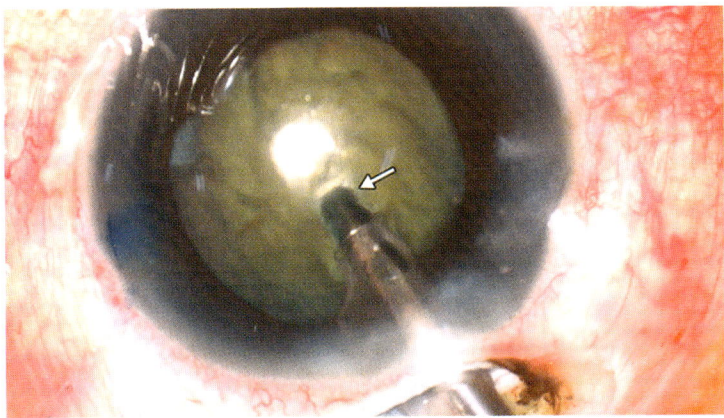

Fig. 9

Result
Bevel down position during trench can give pressure on zonules.

Do's
Trench should be done always in bevel up position of phaco tip.

Observation (Figs. 10A and B)
Change of plane is seen during trench.

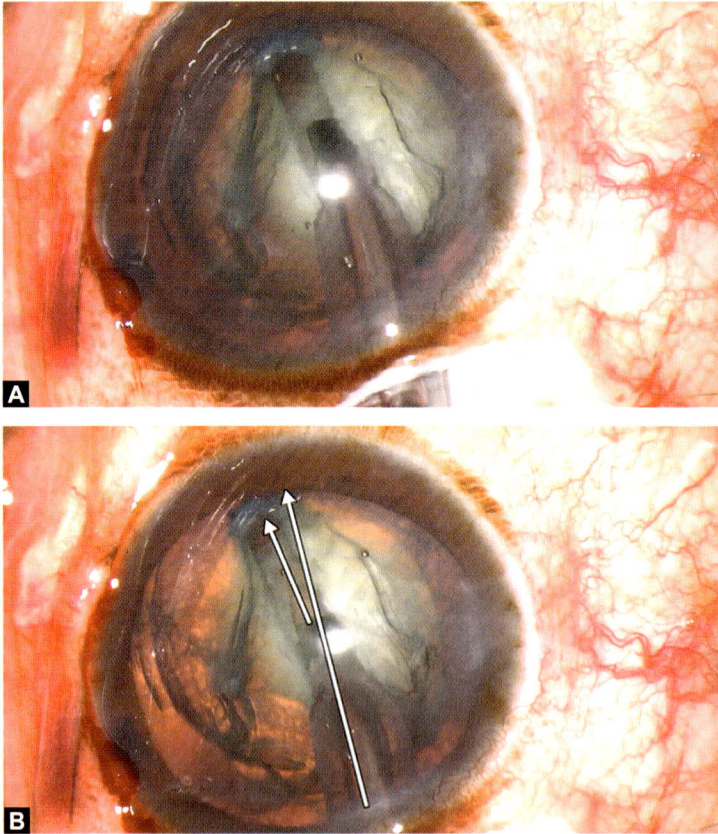

Figs. 10A and B

Results
- Widening of trench can give difficulty for division.
- Multiplanar trench results in debulking of mass which can give rise to difficulty for further step like hold and chop.

Trench 61

Do's
Trench should be done uniplanar except in hard cataract.

Observations (Figs. 11A and B)

During the trench, anterior wall is many times stretched due to:
- Deep anterior chamber
- Deep socket of eye ball
- Pressure on anterior wall of incision during trench
- More angulation of phaco tip during trench
- Use of straight phaco tip.

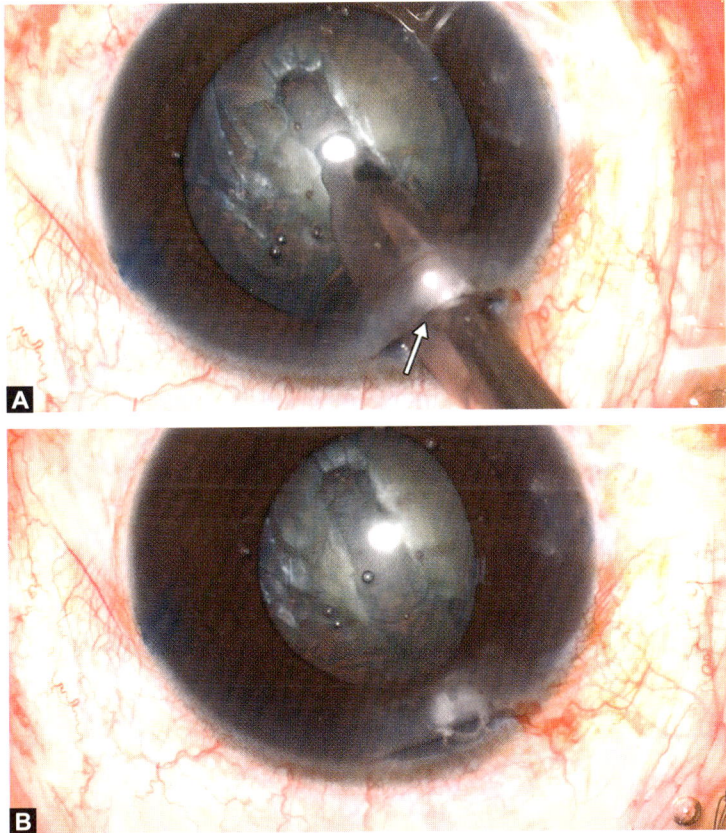

Figs. 11A and B

Results
- Corneal burn is seen due to excessive energy and more rubbing at incision site.

- Architecture of incision can get distorted.
- Vertical stretching of wound is seen.

> **Do's**
> - This is one of the disadvantages of trench.
> - Phaco tip should pass parallel to iris plane during trench.
> - Kelman tip is better option than straight tip to avoid such happenings.
> - Many times, a stitch is needed to close the wound.

Observations (Fig. 12)

- Vertical stretching of the wound due to more angulation of phaco tip during trench.
- Long length of incision will restrict the movement of phaco tip.

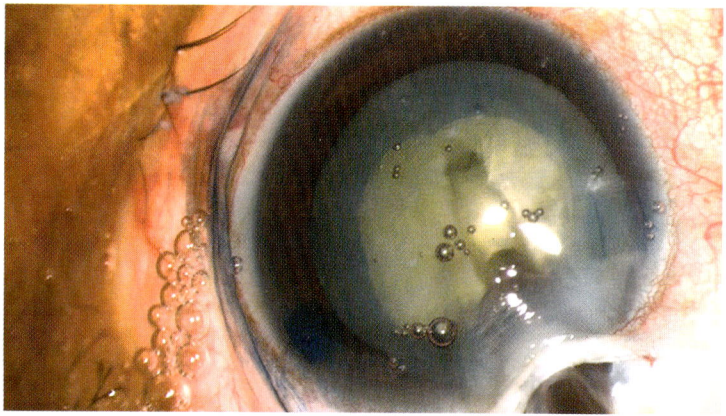

Fig. 12

Result

Cornea can get hazy.

> **Do's**
> - Adequate size of incision with respect to length inside the cornea is important for easy trench.
> - Kelman tip is useful to avoid vertical stretching of wound.

Observations (Figs. 13A and B)

- Trench is going sudden deep in the layers of nucleus.
- Trench is restricted to the center which means inadequate length.
- Uneven anterior chamber as iris is seen in the wound.

- More energy is used than needed.
- Distal end of phaco tip is not visible.

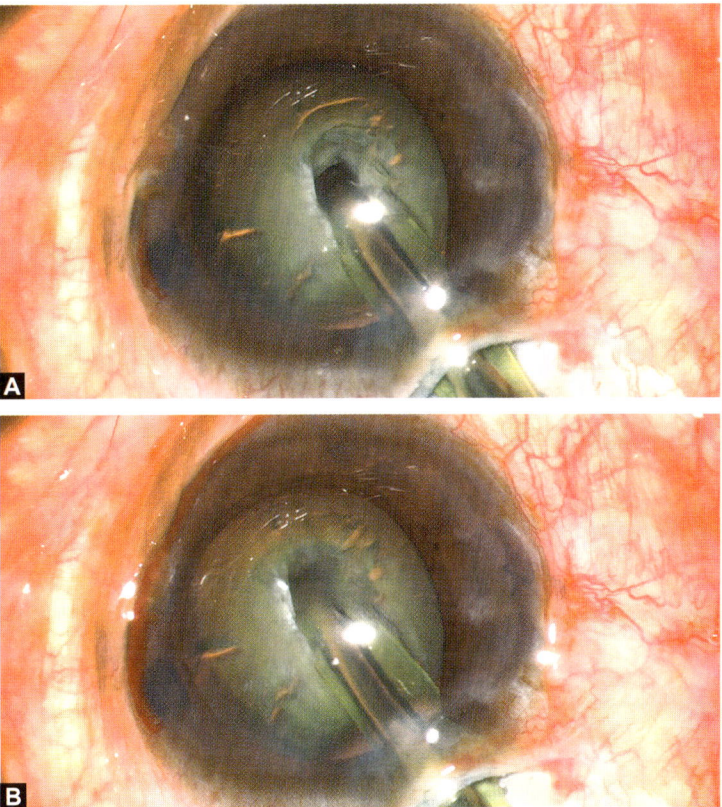

Figs. 13A and B

Results

- Chances of posterior capsule rupture (PCR) with phaco tip can occur.
- Injury to iris or corneal burn can occur.

Do's
- *Trench should be done layer by layer and adequate length.*
- *Anterior chamber should be normal before start of trench.*
- *Angulation of the phaco tip should be parallel to iris plane.*
- *Energy used should be adequate with uniform speed.*

Observations (Figs. 14A to F)

- Sleeve is stucked in first few photographs.
- Trench is going on and suddenly sleeve is released.
- With more pressure to release the sleeve, surgeon is reaching to the periphery (Beyond capsulorhexis) and sculpts soft part of nucleus or epinucleus.

Result

Trench in soft part of nucleus or epinucleus can cause PCR.

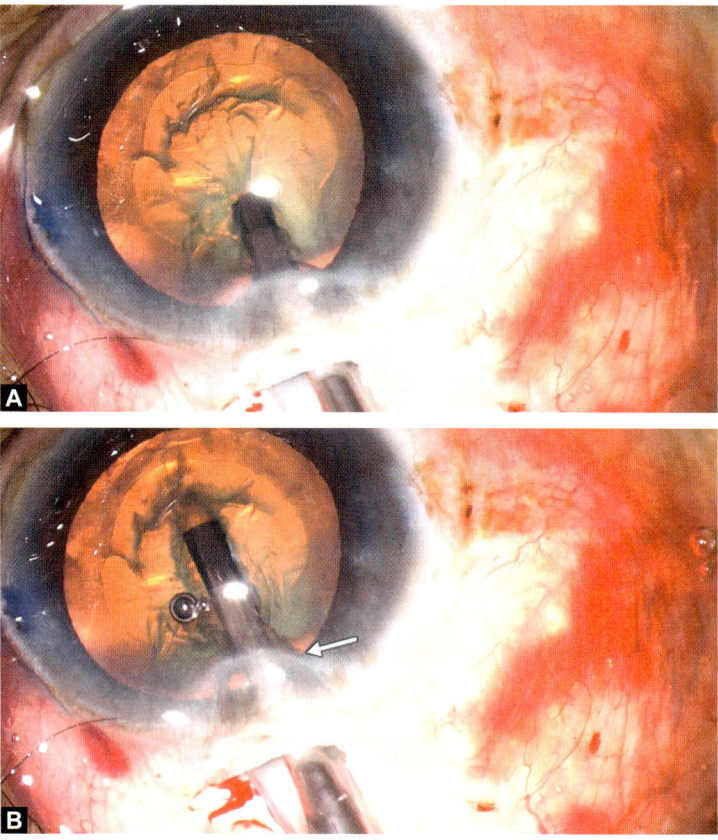

Figs. 14A and B

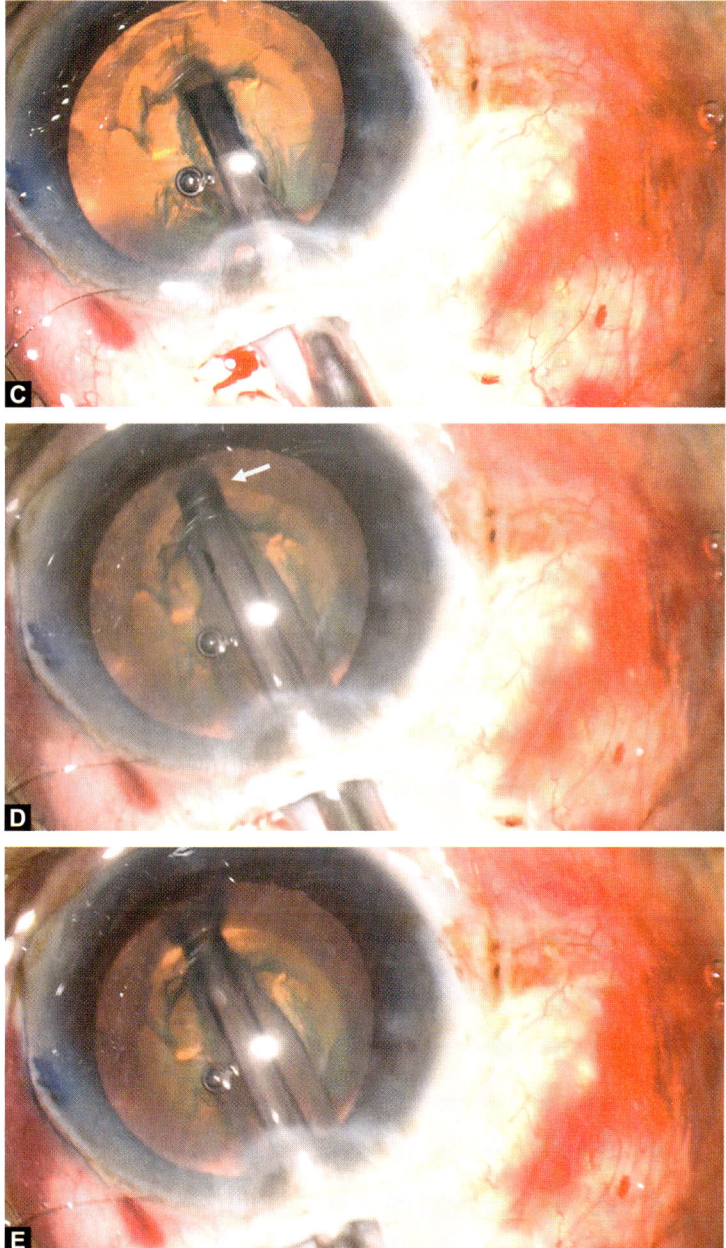

Figs. 14C to E

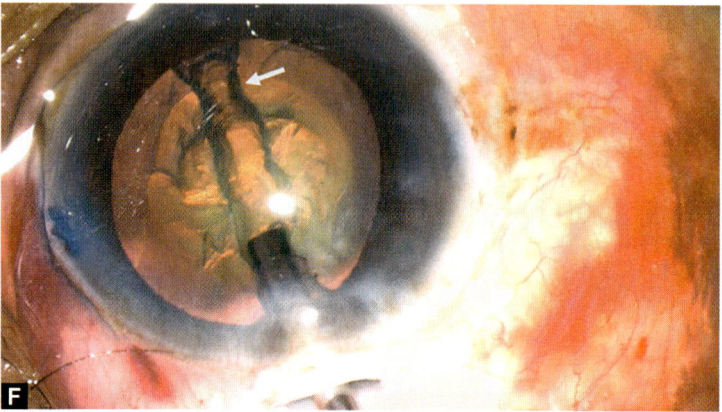

Fig. 14F

Do's
- During trench, such situation can occur.
- Generally do not cross capsulorhexis during trench.
- Avoid the trench in epinucleus.

Observations (Figs. 15A and B)
- Trench is unequal.
- In unequal trench, surgeon unable to do deep trench, as posterior capsule is near to phaco tip.

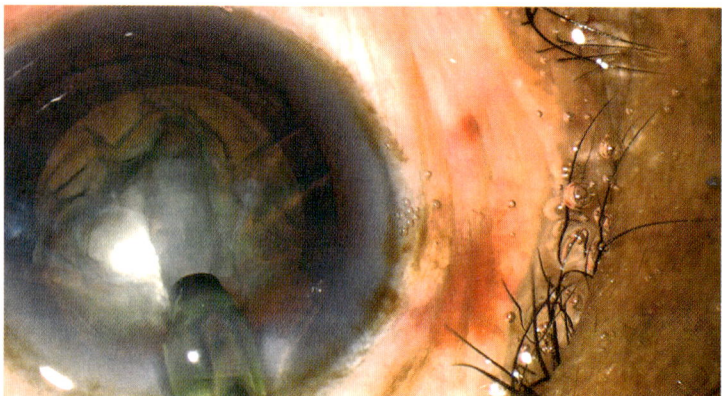

Fig. 15A

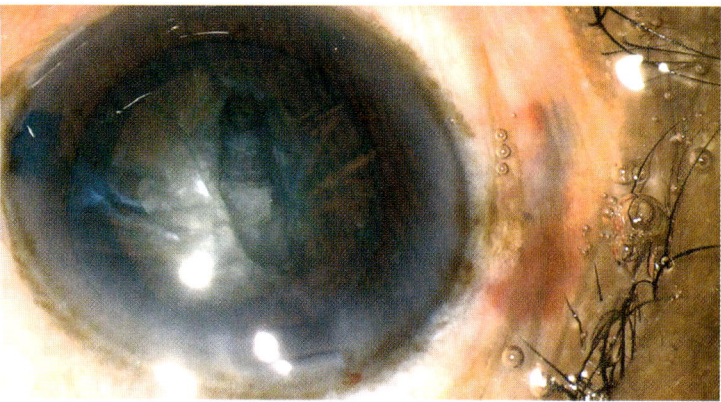

Fig. 15B

Results
- Unequal trench is difficult to divide.
- Unequal division will lead difficulty for further step of hold and chop.

Do's
Central trench of nucleus is important prerequisite for better division and further nucleus management.

CHAPTER 5

Division of Nucleus

INTRODUCTION

- Division is most crucial step in phaco surgery.
- Instruments which are needed are dialer, chopper, phaco tip, and prechopper.
- Handling of these instruments during this step is really learning process.
- Change of plane from incision site to base of nucleus is really needed to consider in this step.

DIVISION BY DIALER AND CHOPPER

Observations (Figs. 1A and B)

- Division is done by dialer and chopper.
- Difficulty to pass chopper through side port incision.
- Iris is shifted towards incision.
- Shallow or uneven anterior chamber.

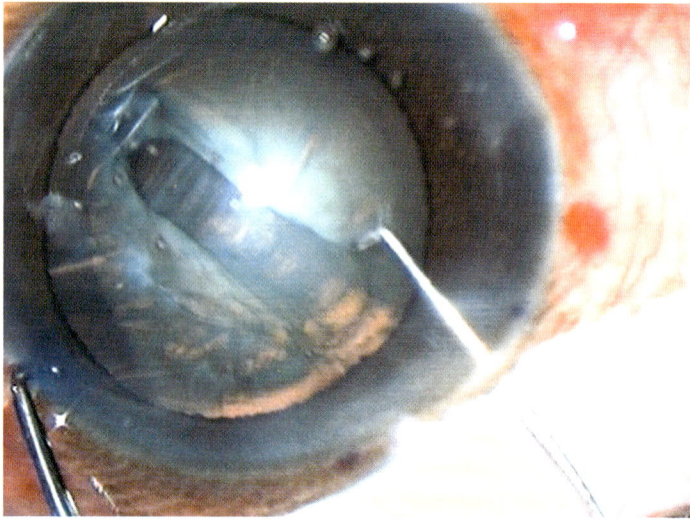

Fig. 1A

Division of Nucleus

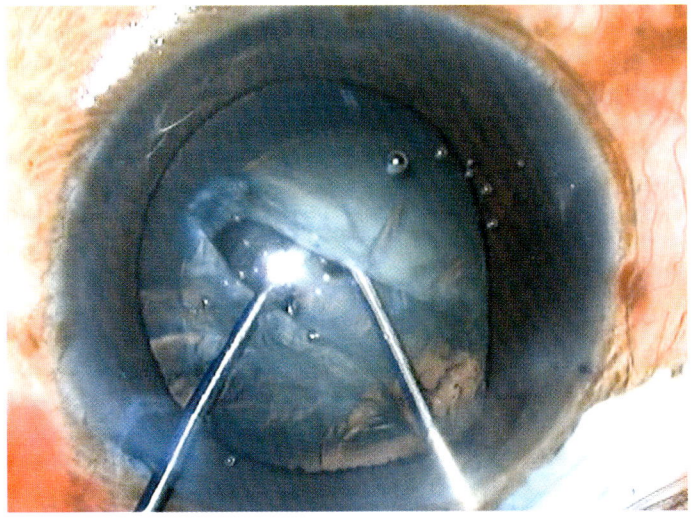

Fig. 1B

Result

Slow entry and movement of dialer leaks the wound.

> **Do's**
> Adequate angulation and movement of dialer and chopper is first step to learn division.

Observation (Figs. 2A to C)

Direction of the chopper is wrongly placed.

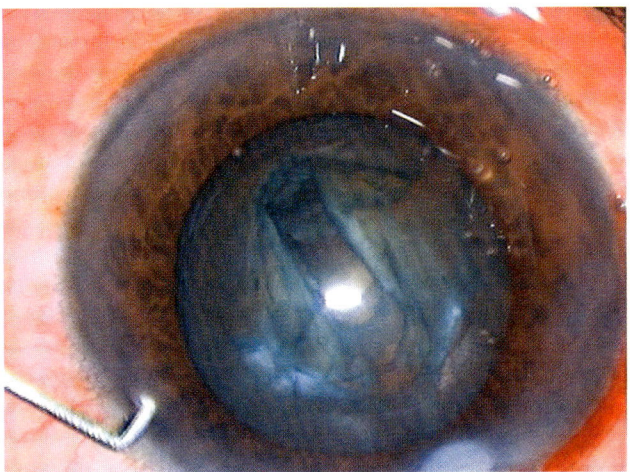

Fig. 2A

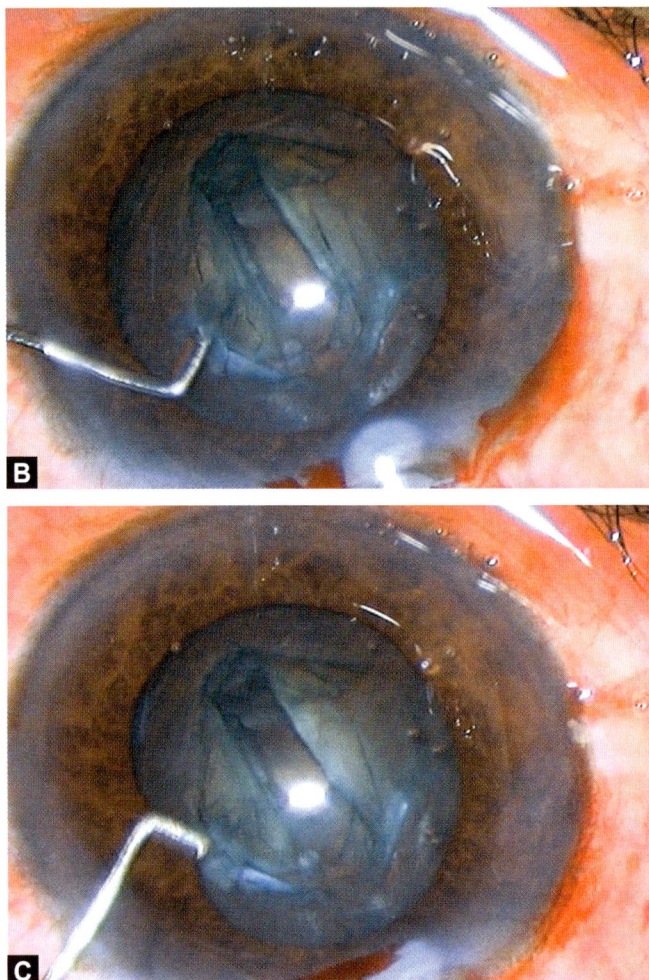

Figs. 2B and C

Result

During change in position, iris is getting injured.

Do's
Placement of the chopper should be horizontal with tip directed towards main incision.

Observations

- Chopper placed vertically (Fig. 3A).

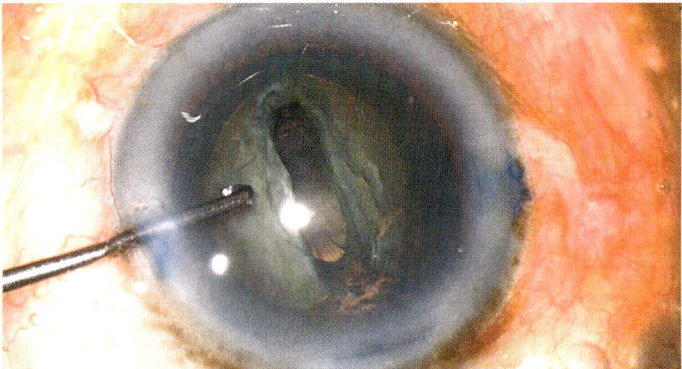

Fig. 3A

- Chopper placed obliquely (Fig. 3B).

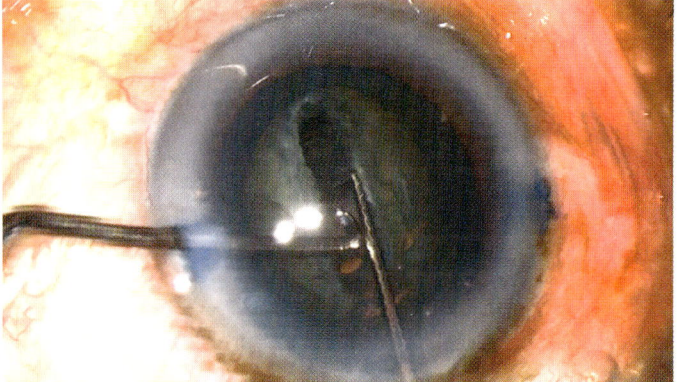

Fig. 3B

- Chopper is not visualized clearly (Fig. 3C).
- Pressure is on side port incision by chopper.

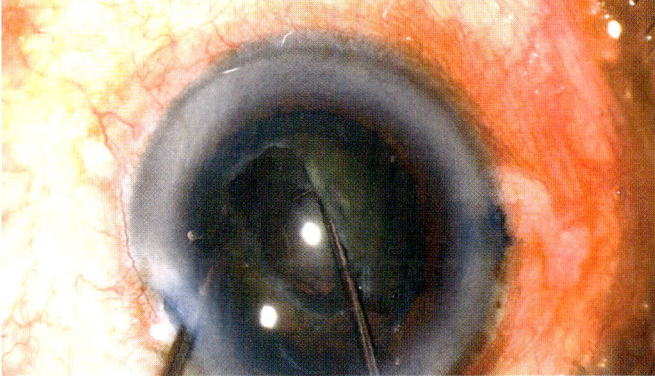

Fig. 3C

- Both dialer and chopper ends are not visible (Fig. 3D).
- Chopper and dialer placed at different planes, i.e. chopper at superficial and dialer at plane of nucleus.

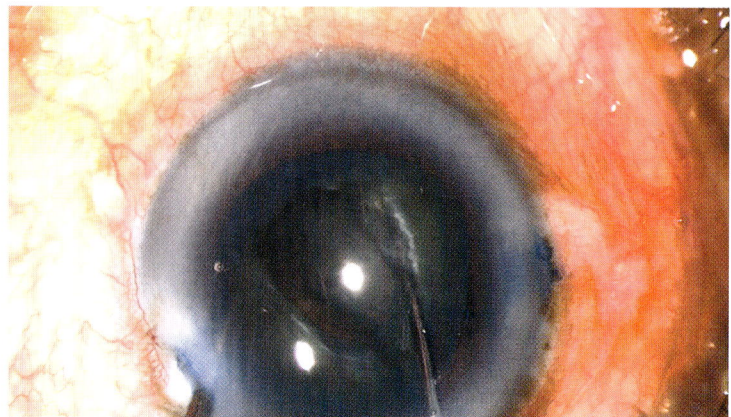

Fig. 3D

Result

Uneven division.

Observations (Fig. 3E)

- Chopper and dialer are superficially placed.
- More force is needed to complete division.

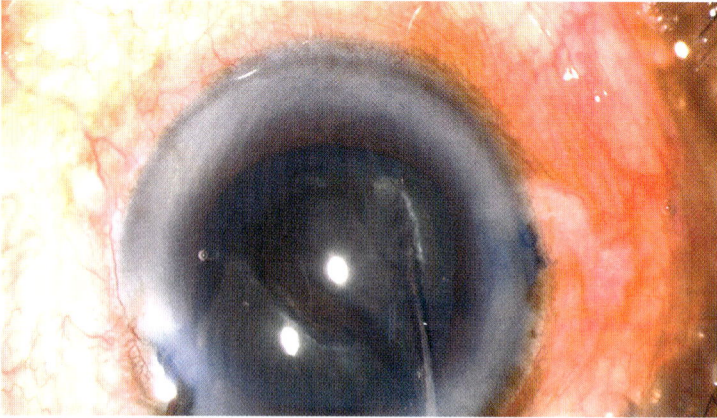

Fig. 3E

Result

Pressure on zonules.

Observation (Fig. 3F)

As both instruments are placed superficially, instruments have to pass more distance to separate two halves of nucleus.

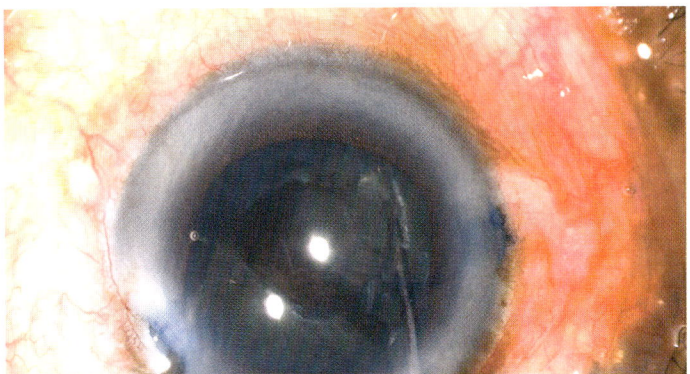

Fig. 3F

Result

This maneuver can give pressure on zonules.

Do's (Figs. 3A to F)
- Both instruments should be in one plane and preferably in the bulk or deeper plane of nucleus.
- Equal force is required for division.

AFTER DIVISION, WHILE INSTRUMENTS ARE COMING OUT—FOLLOWING POINTS ARE NOTED:

Observations
- Chopper is placed vertically down (Fig. 4A).

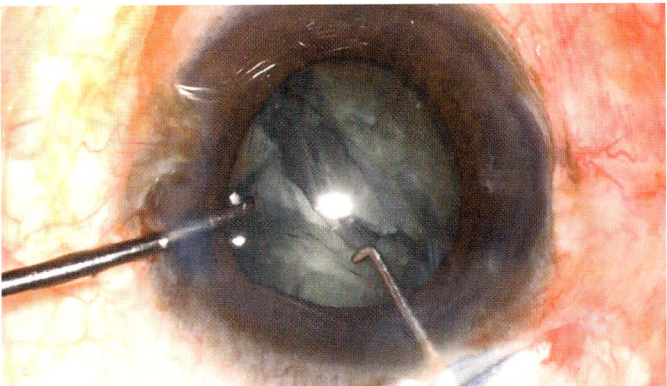

Fig. 4A

- Chopper is hitting iris and cornea (Fig. 4B).

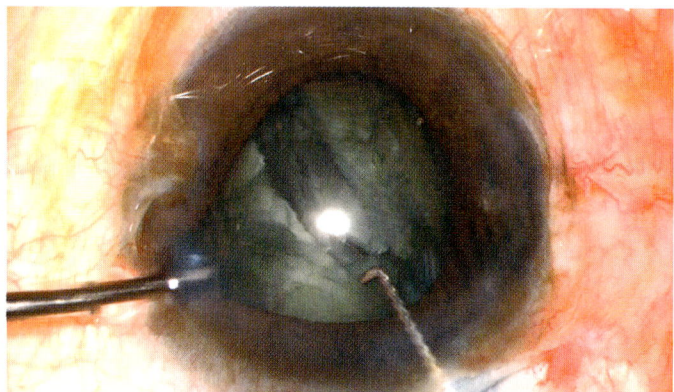

Fig. 4B

Observations (Fig. 4C)

- Chopper is stucked in side port incision which can stretch cornea (Fig. 4C).
- Dialer can touch iris.

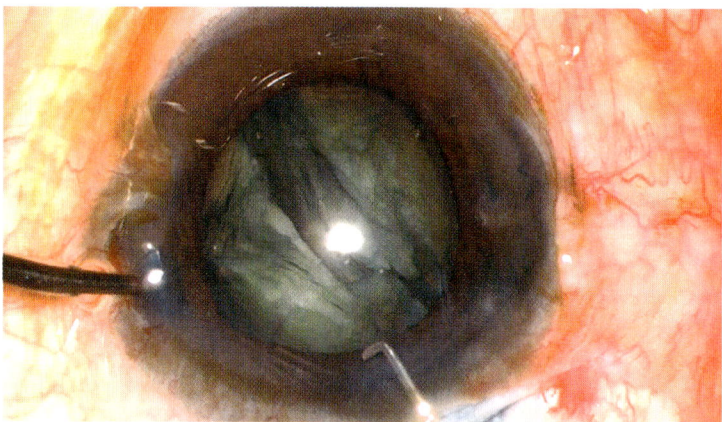

Fig. 4C

Result

Cornea, iris, and anterior capsule can get damaged.

Do's (Figs. 4A to C)
- *Passing both instruments, dialer and chopper, in and out is an art.*
- *Place these instruments horizontal during passing in and out.*
- *These instruments are working vertical or oblique position during division.*

Observations (Figs. 5A and B)

- In both cases, division is complete but instruments (dialer and chopper or prechopper) used for division are placed superficially.
- Distance of separation is more during division.
- More force is used for division.

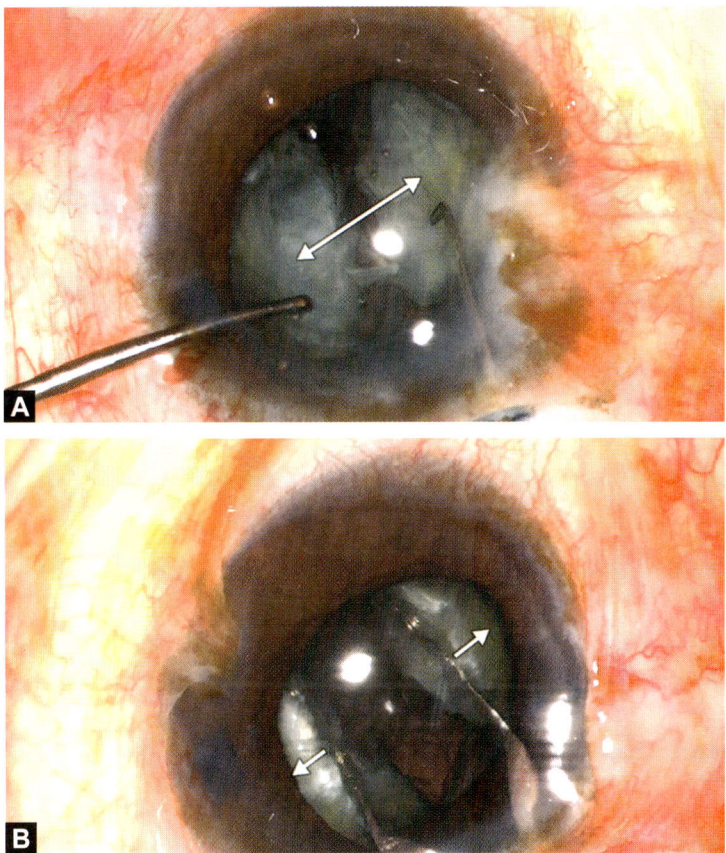

Figs. 5A and B

Results
- Cracking the posterior plate of nucleus is difficult.
- Pressure on zonules which leads to zonular dialysis.

> **Do's**
> Division should be done in bulk or at posterior plane (deep) with adequate force.

Observations (Figs. 6A and B)

- Dialer and chopper are superficial.
- More pressure with dialer and chopper during procedure.

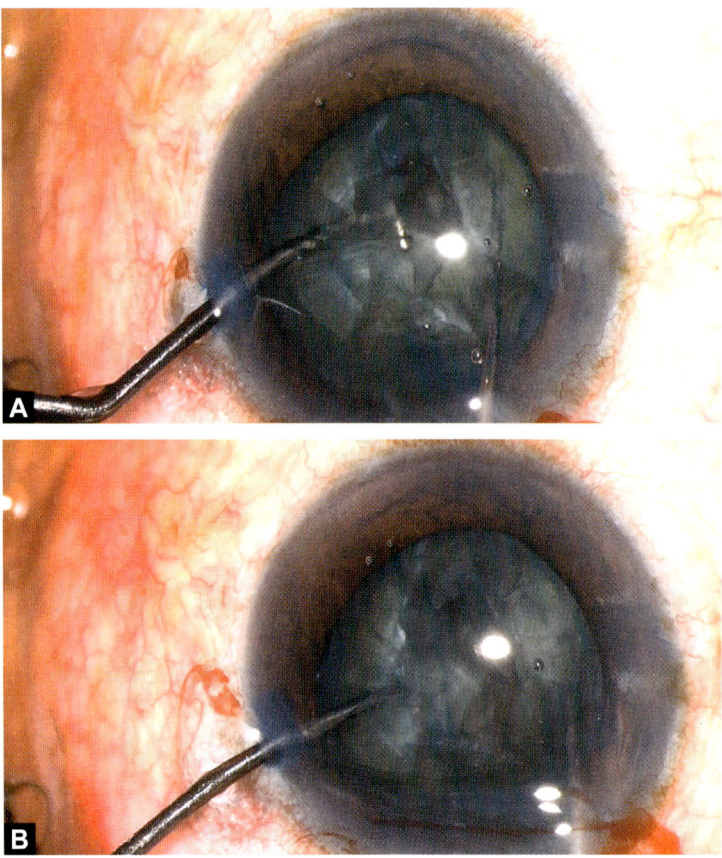

Figs. 6A and B

Results

- Folds on cornea seen.
- Visualization is hampered.

Do's
Handling of instruments should be smooth and working at correct plane.

Division of Nucleus

Observations (Figs. 7A and B)

- Dialer and chopper used for confirmation of superior division.
- More pressure by chopper.
- End of dialer is not visible.
- Anterior chamber is shallow.

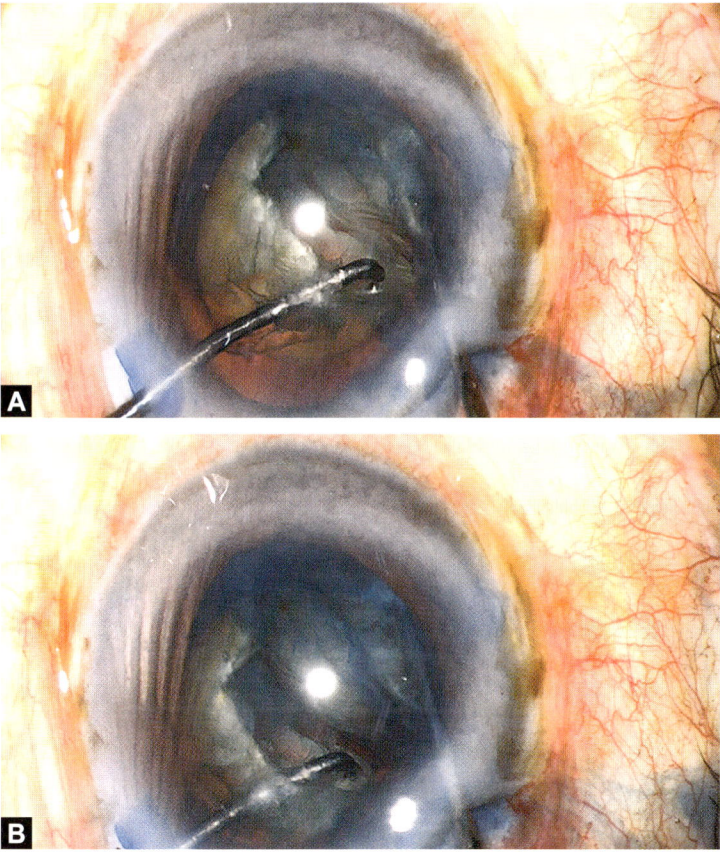

Figs. 7A and B

Result

Shallow anterior chamber is one of the hurdles for division which can give stress on zonules and causing injury to iris or cornea.

Do's (Figs. 7A and B)
- *Pressure by instruments should be avoided during this step.*
- *Instruments should be visible throughout the procedure.*
- *Deepening of anterior chamber is must.*

DIVISION BY TOSHNIWAL PRECHOPPER (ASICO 4187)

Observation (Figs. 8A and B)

Oblique entry of prechopper.

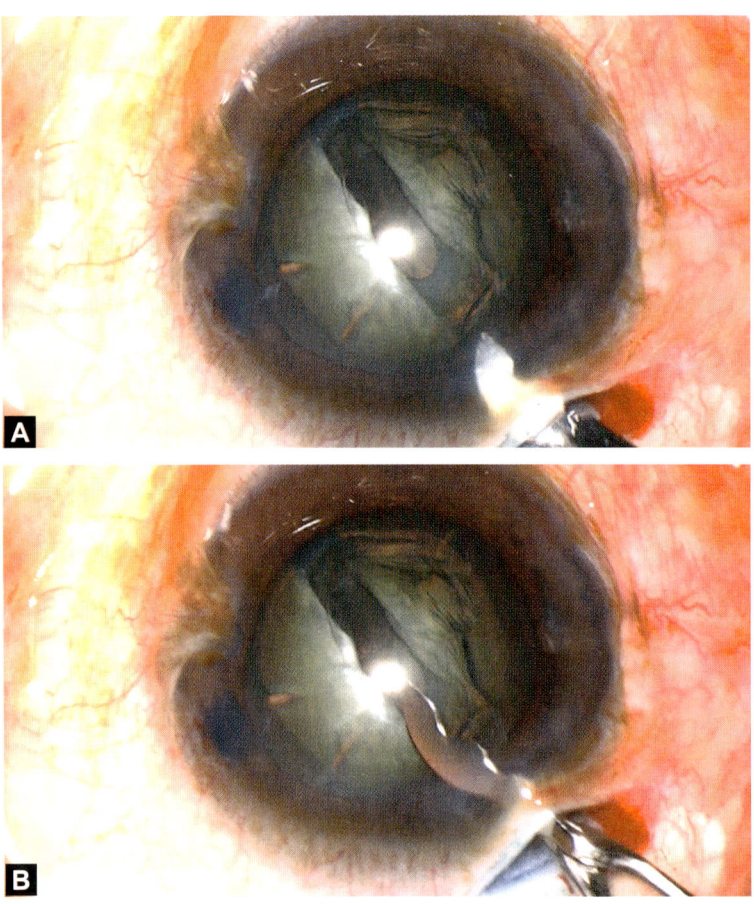

Figs. 8A and B

Observation (Figs. 8C and D)

Prechopper is placed away from center.

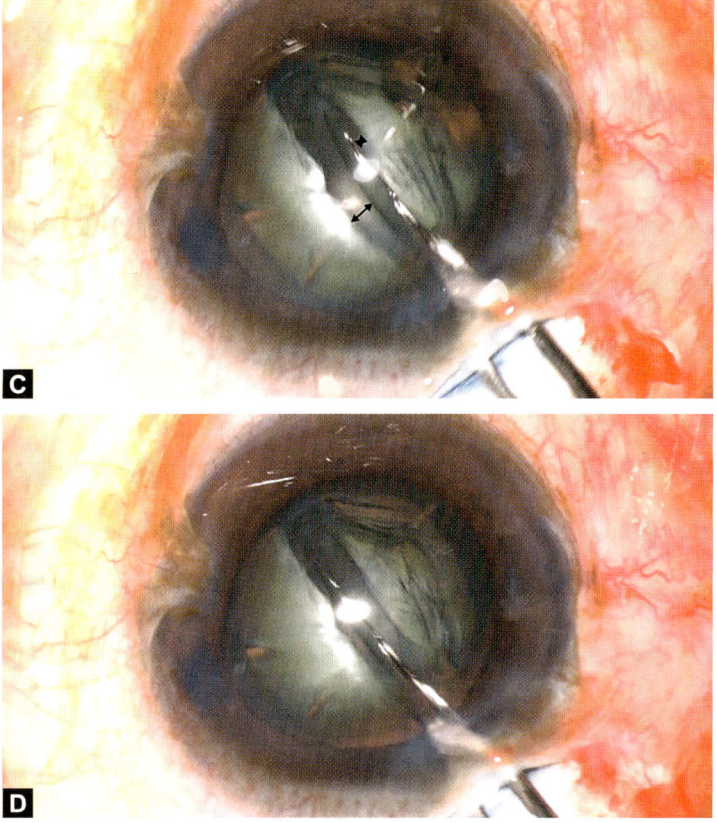

Figs. 8C and D

Observations (Figs. 8E and F)

- Prechopper is dividing nucleus in the anterior plane of the nucleus.
- More pressure is needed to divide the nucleus.
- Distance between two plates of prechopper is more.

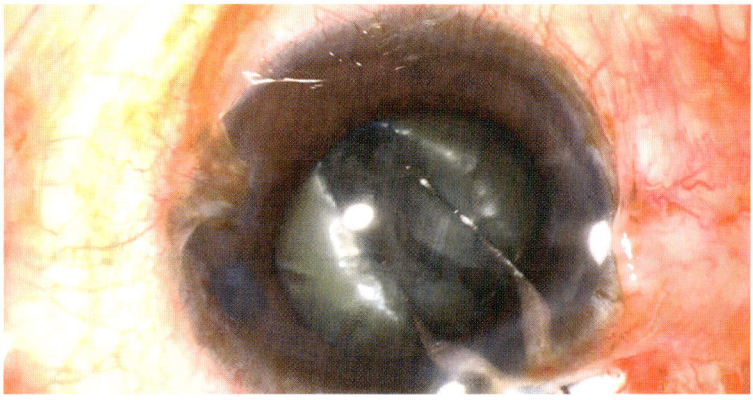

Fig. 8E

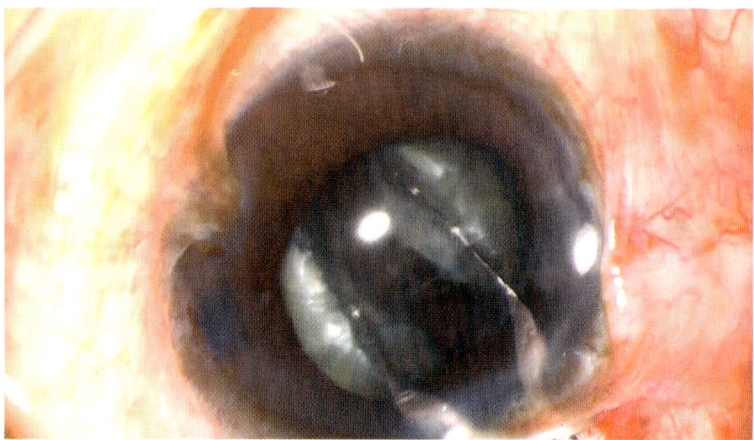

Fig. 8F

Results

- Injury to cornea or iris can occur (Figs. 8A and B)
- Division of nucleus will be unequal (Figs. 8C and D)
- Pressure on zonules can occur (Figs. 8E and F)

Do's (Figs. 8A to F)
- Prechopper should pass horizontally in and out of anterior chamber to avoid injury to cornea and iris.
- Placement of the prechopper blade is in bevel-up position in the center of groove by touching the base of trench.

Observation (Figs. 9A to D)

Trench is superficial.

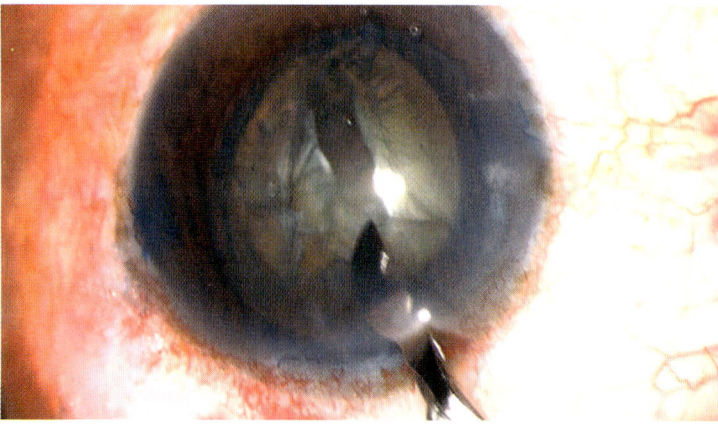

Fig. 9A

Division of Nucleus 81

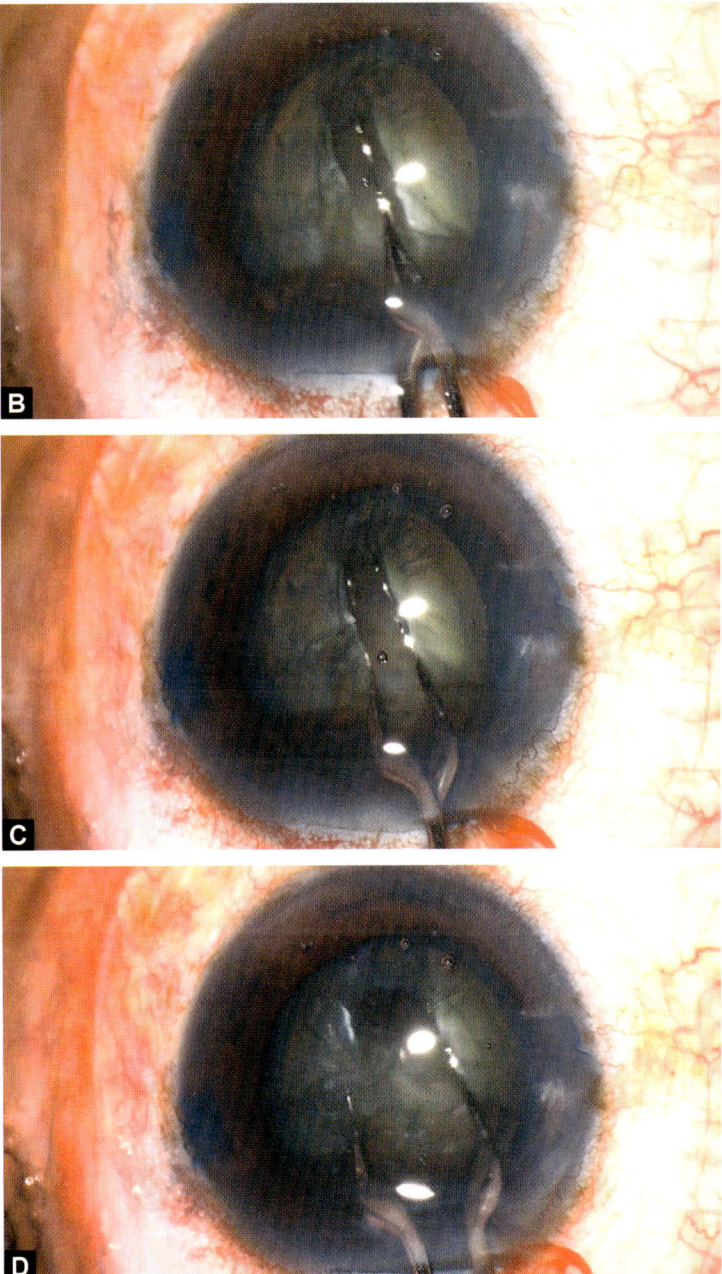

Figs. 9B to D

Result

Division is difficult with prechopper also.

Do's
- *Proper depth of trench is the most important prerequisite for division.*
- *Repeat the trench till it reaches the proper depth for adequate division (More than 1/2 to 2/3rd of the nucleus).*

Observation (Figs. 10A and B)

Prechopper is placed obliquely in the groove.

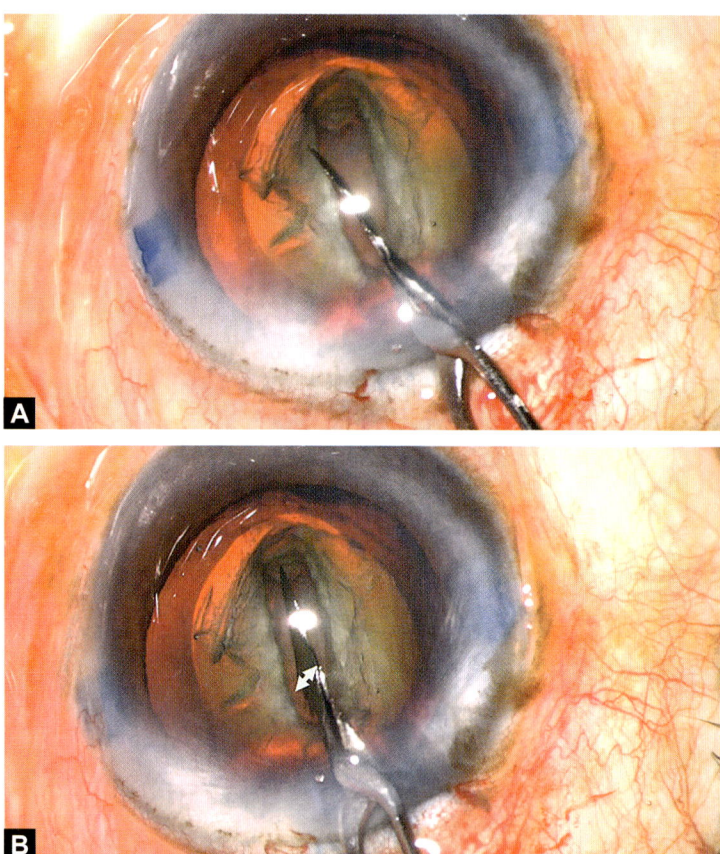

Figs. 10A and B

Result

Division is unequal.

Do's
Prechopper should be placed vertical and straight deep in the center for better division.

DIVISION BY PHACO TIP AND CHOPPER

Observation (Figs. 11A to C)

Trench is attempted by phaco tip and chopper.

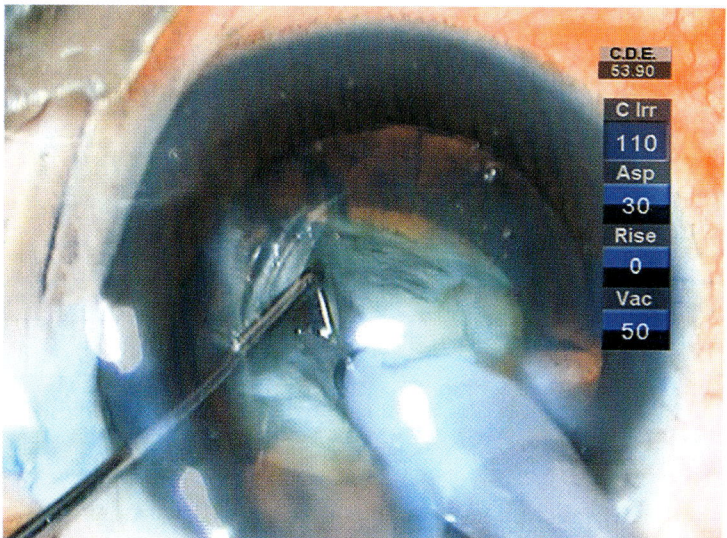

Fig. 11A

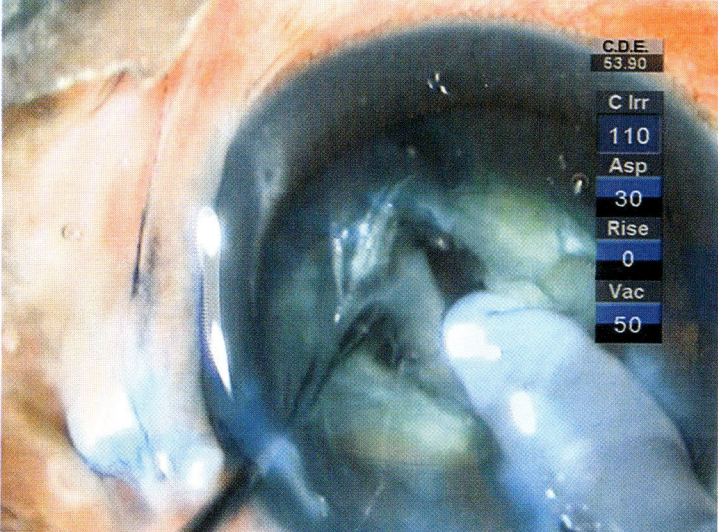

Fig. 11B

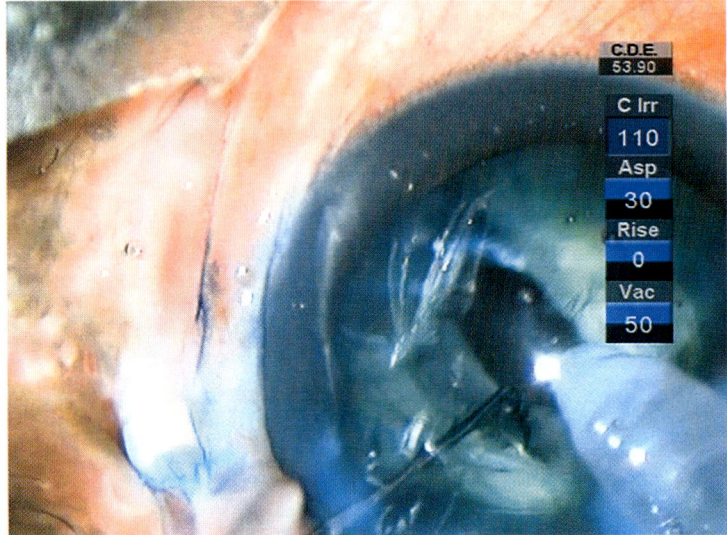

Fig. 11C

Result

Many times, division is unequal due to use of uneven instruments.

Do's
To avoid unequal division, author prefers using dialer and chopper or Toshniwal prechopper.

A CASE SERIES BY DIALER AND CHOPPER IN ONE CASE (FIGS. 12A TO I)

Observations

- Trench is relatively superficial (so expect difficult division).
- More pressure is needed to divide.
- Plane of dialer and chopper are at a different level.
- Both the hemispheres have turned to superior and inferior position.

Division of Nucleus 85

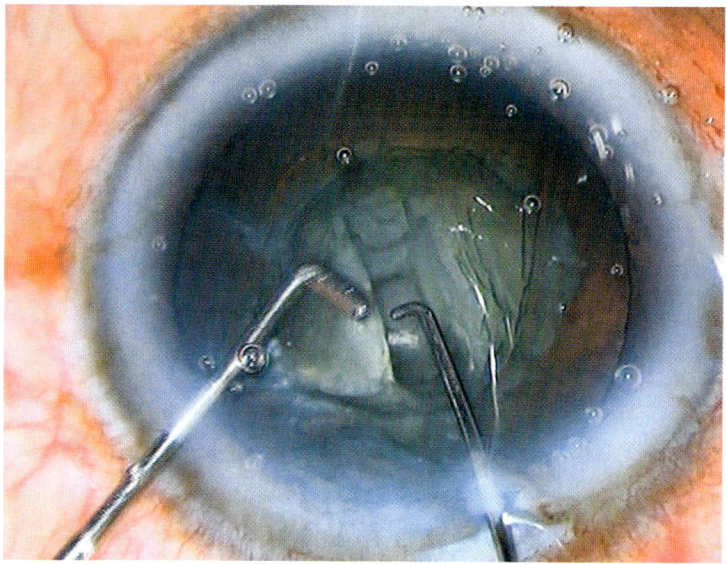

Fig. 12A

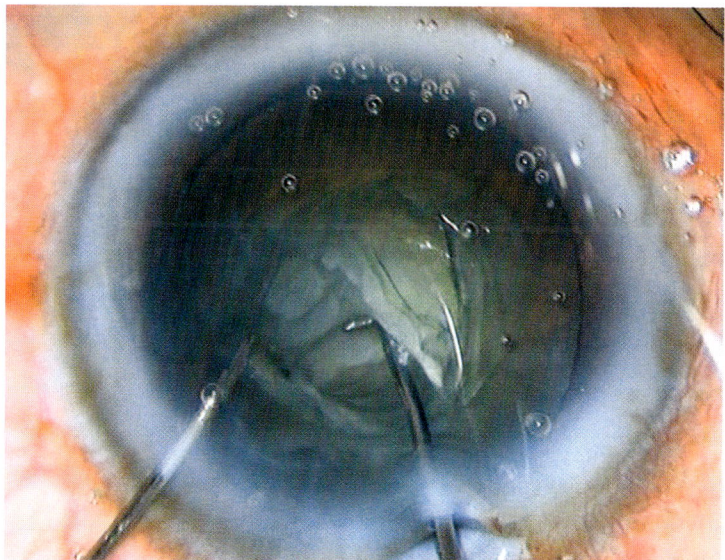

Fig. 12B

86 Do's and Don'ts in Phaco Surgery: Text and Atlas

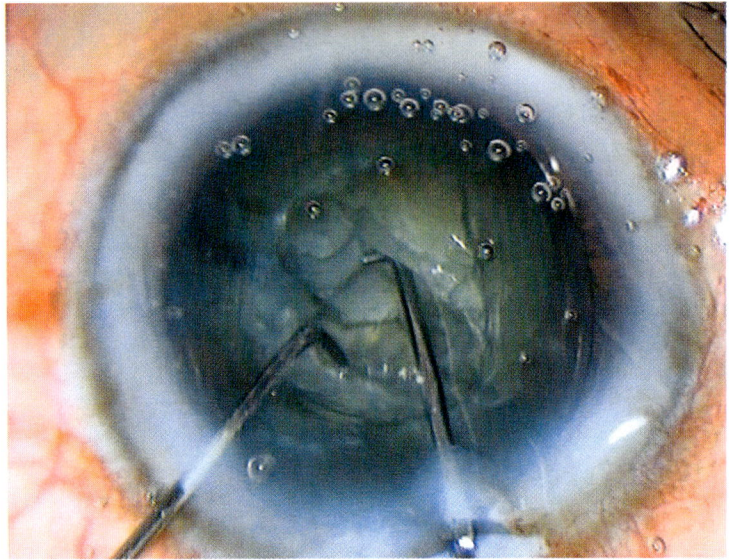

Fig. 12C

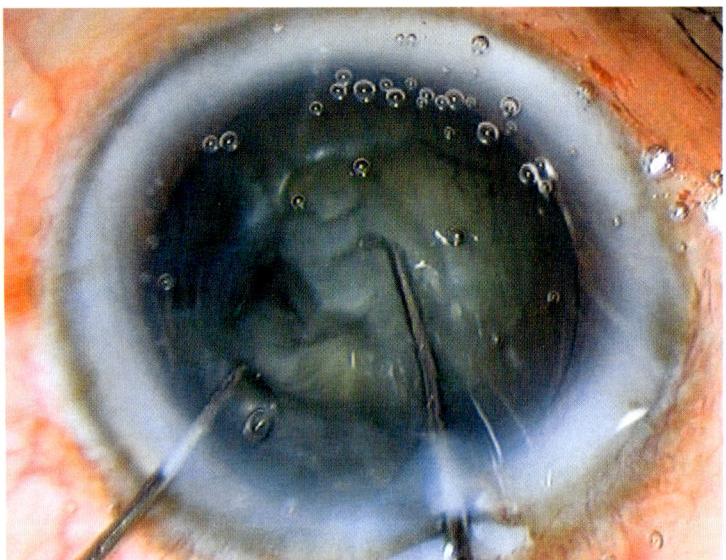

Fig. 12D

Division of Nucleus

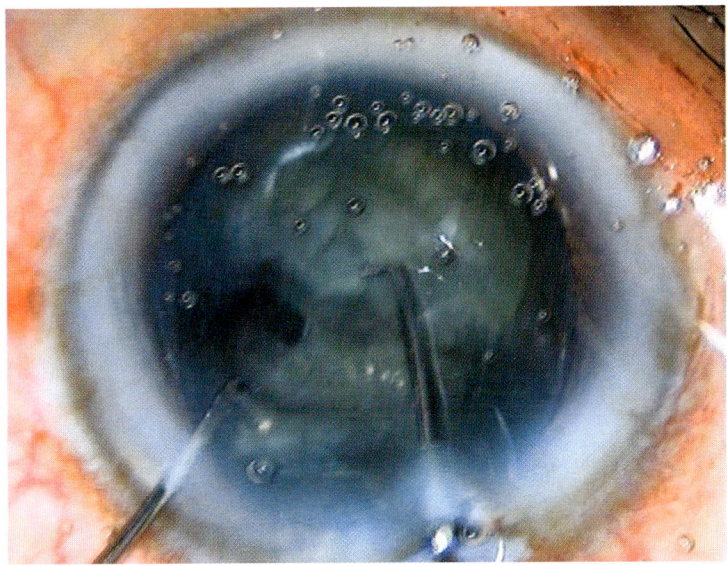

Fig. 12E

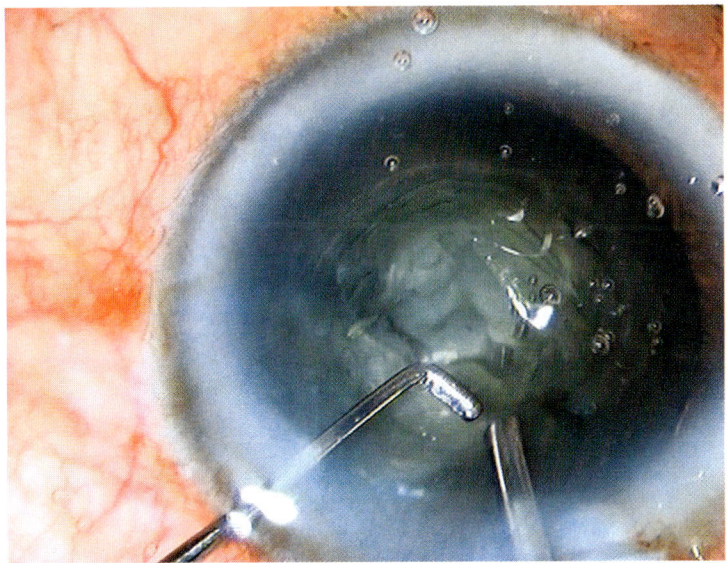

Fig. 12F

88 Do's and Don'ts in Phaco Surgery: Text and Atlas

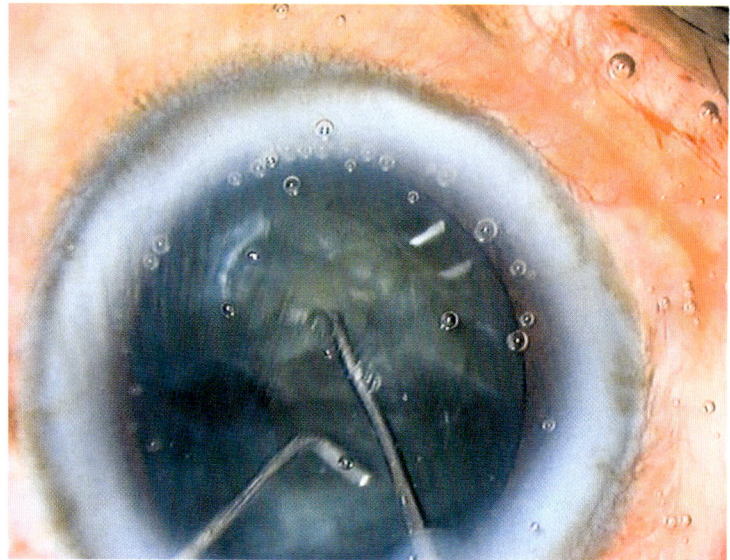

Fig. 12G

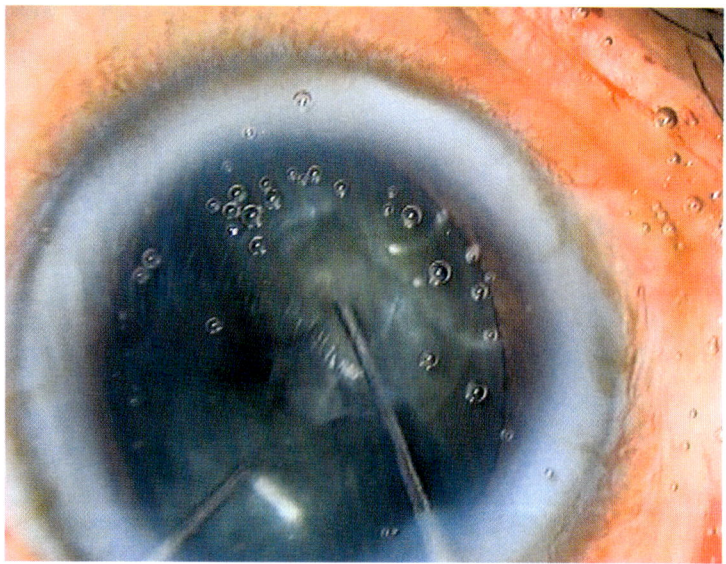

Fig. 12H

Division of Nucleus

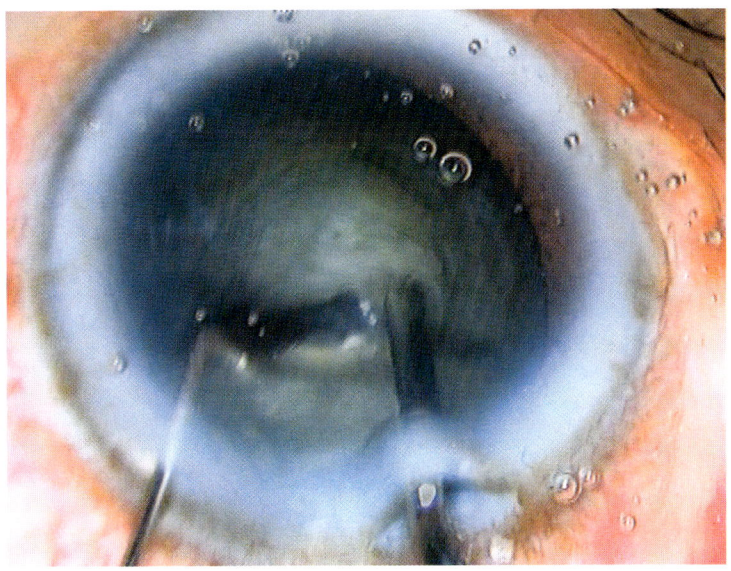

Fig. 12I

Results

- Division seems to be difficult in this position.
- Shallowing of anterior chamber can occur.

> *Do's*
> - *Deep uniplanar trench is the most important prerequisite for division.*
> - *Both the instruments, dialer and chopper, should be placed in the groove.*
> - *Equal force with wrist movement in one plane is needed to divide in this situation.*
> - *As superior-inferior position is not ideal for division, surgeon has to change the position of halves of the nucleus as right and left or lateral and medial.*

A CASE SERIES OF SHALLOW TRENCH

Observations (Figs. 13A to H)

- Shallow anterior chamber.
- Trench is superficial.
- More pressure is needed for division—anterior chamber gets shallower—difficulty for division continues (vicious cycle).

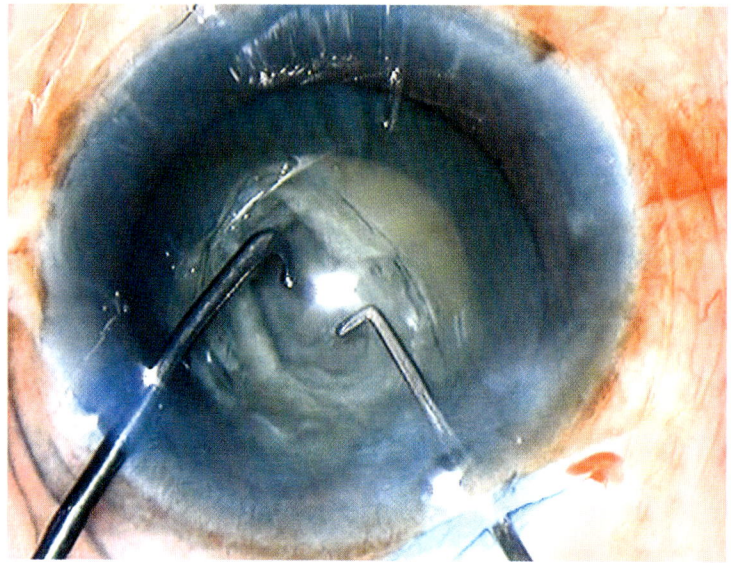

Fig. 13A

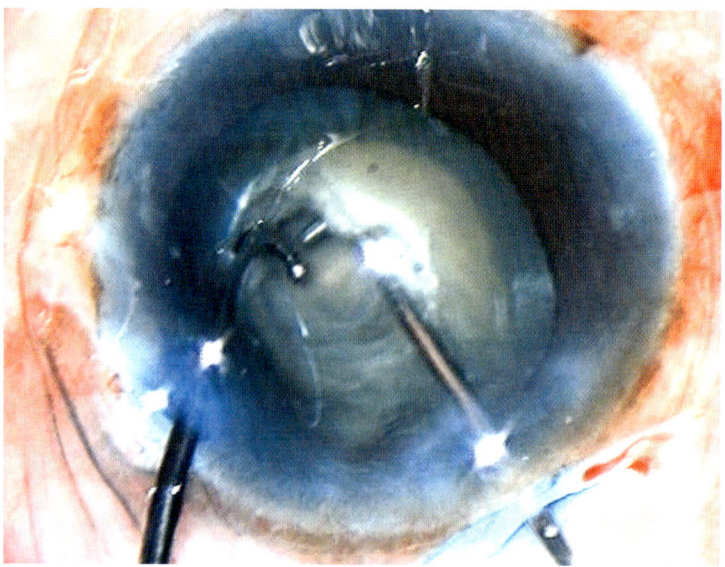

Fig. 13B

Division of Nucleus

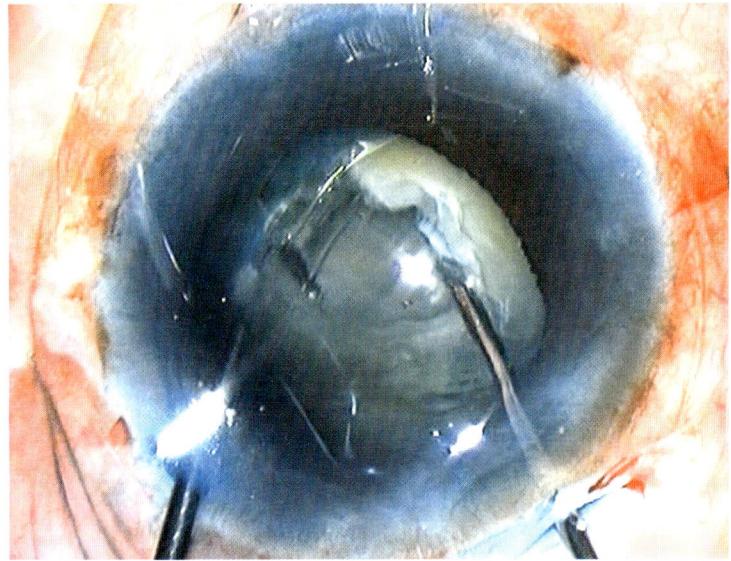

Fig. 13C

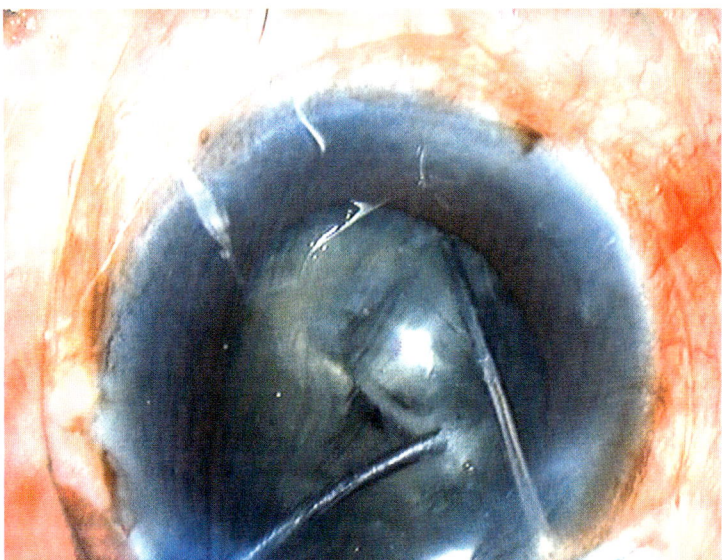

Fig. 13D

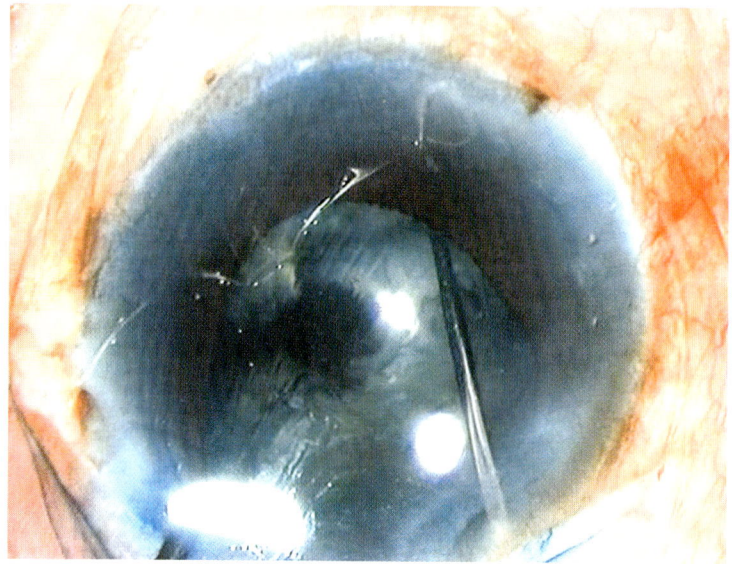

Fig. 13E

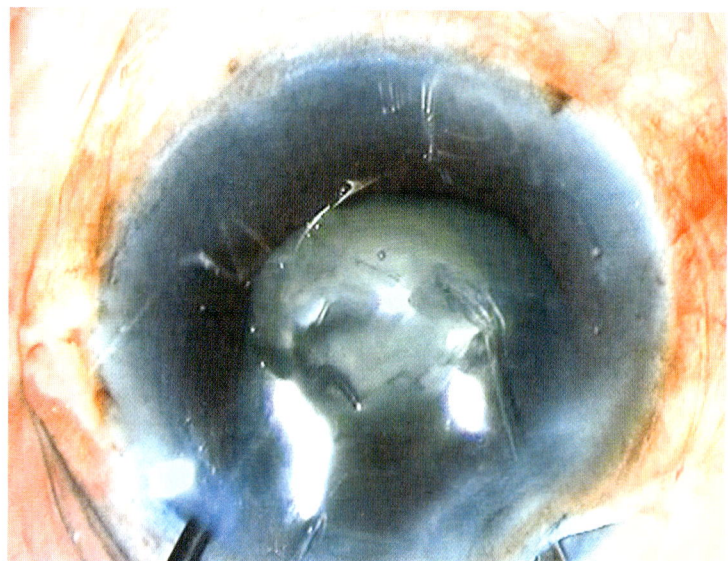

Fig. 13F

Division of Nucleus

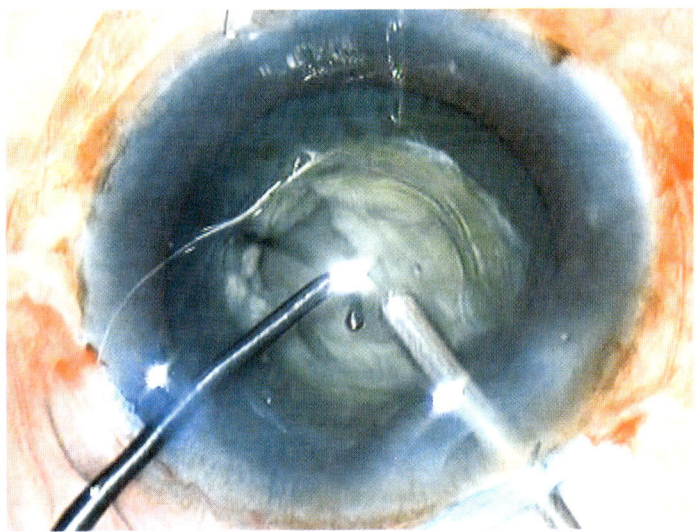

Fig. 13G

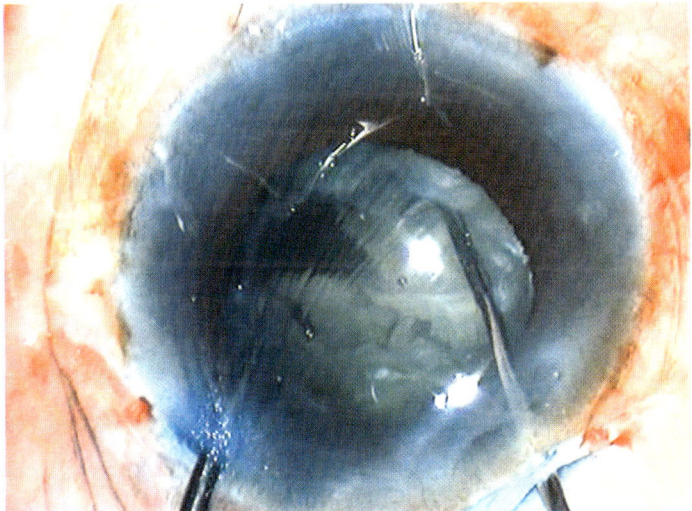

Fig. 13H

Result

Complete division is difficult in this situation.

Do's
- *Adequate depth of trench and maintaining normal anterior chamber during procedure is important for division.*

Observation (Figs. 14A to F)

Division by dialer and chopper in acrossed way.

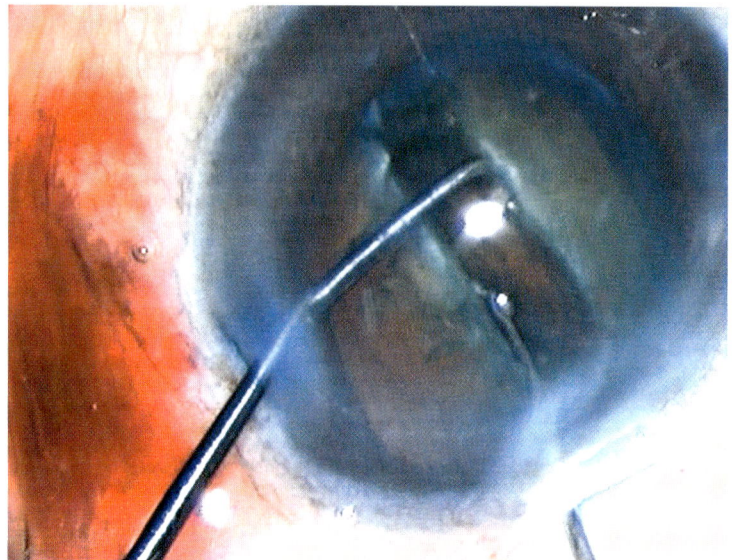

Fig. 14A

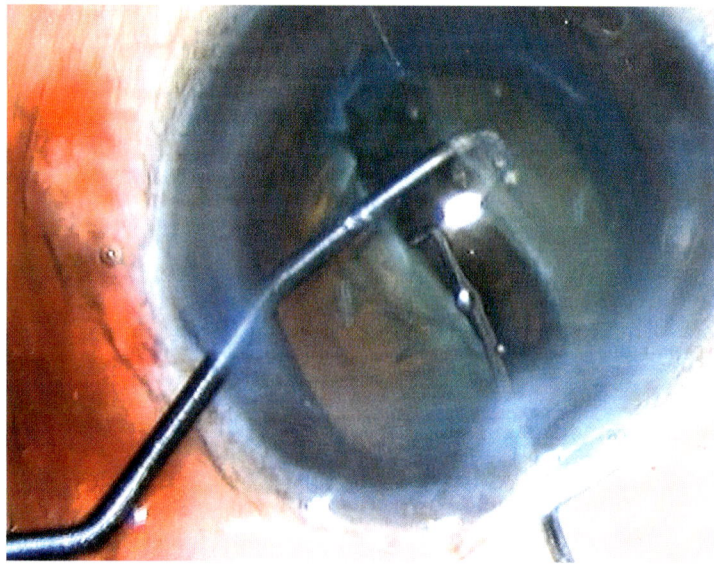

Fig. 14B

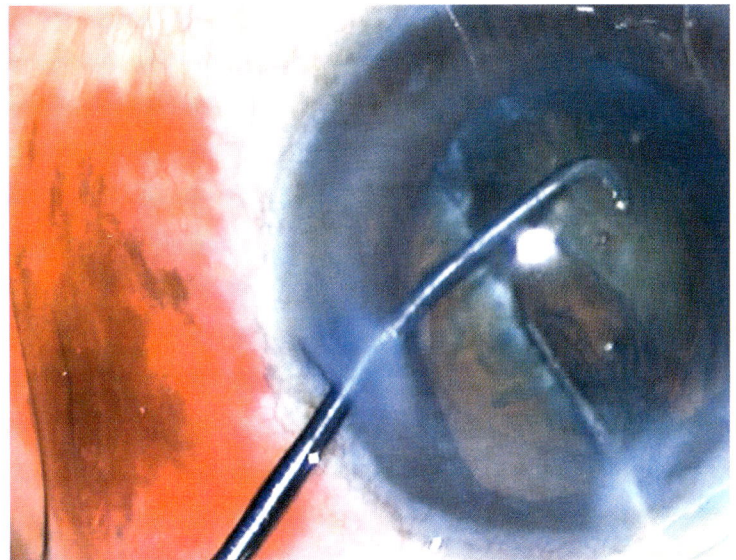

Fig. 14C

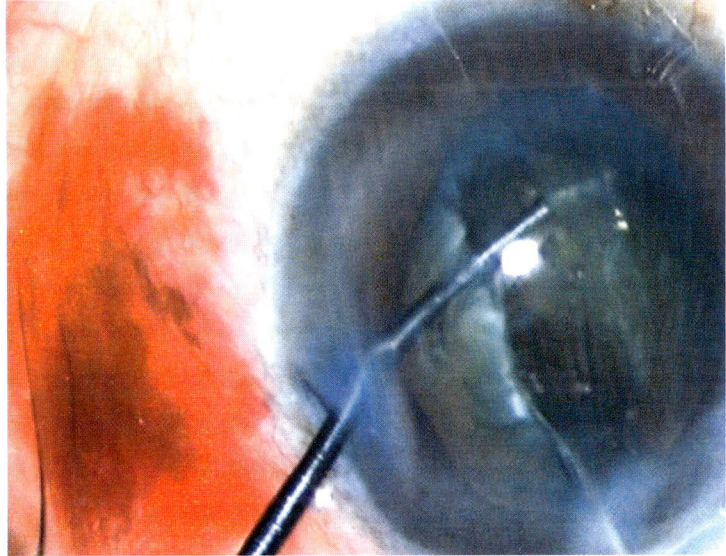

Fig. 14D

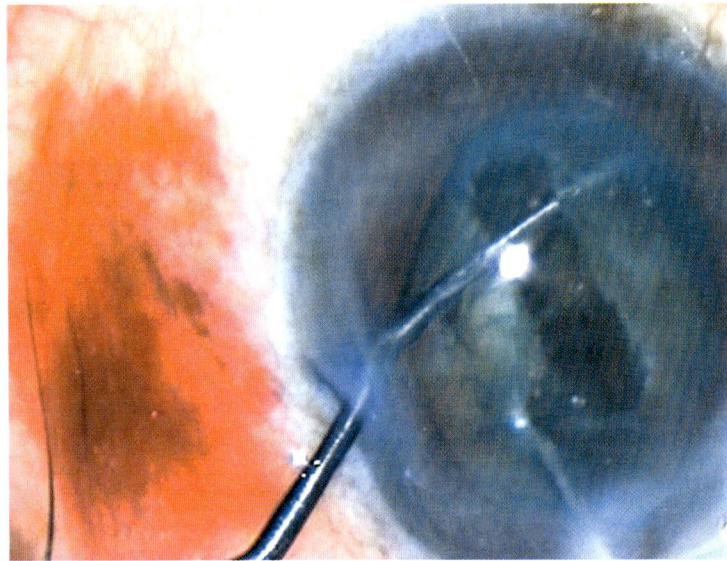

Fig. 14E

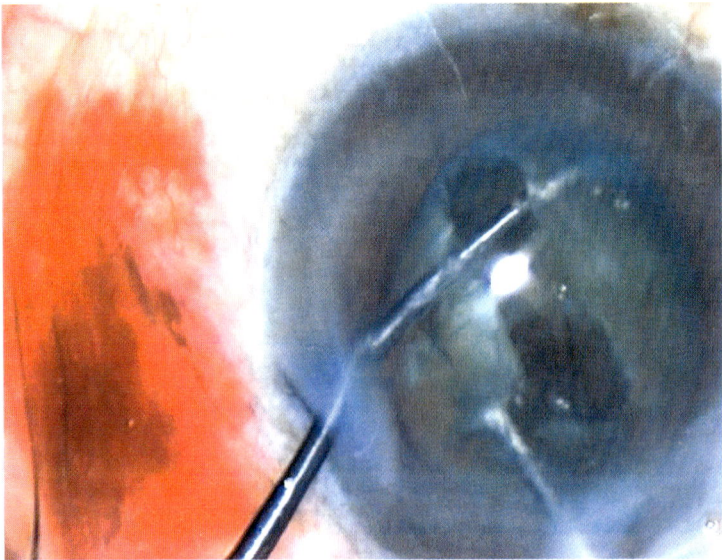

Fig. 14F

Result

Division may be difficult as instruments are not in one plane.

Do's
Division should be done by placing the instrument in one plane.

CHAPTER 6

Hold and Chop of Nucleus

INTRODUCTION

- This is one of the important steps of nucleus management.
- Understanding of vacuum and flow rate is important.
- Phaco tip angulation with respect to nucleus is a key factor for success of this step.
- Handling of chopper is a learning process.
- Correlation of chopper and phaco tip is important and should be in conceptual way.

PLACEMENT OF PHACO TIP IN HOLD AND CHOP

Observations (Fig. 1)

- Attempt of hold in superficial part of nucleus.
- There is a trench-like picture during hold.
- Energy used is more than needed.

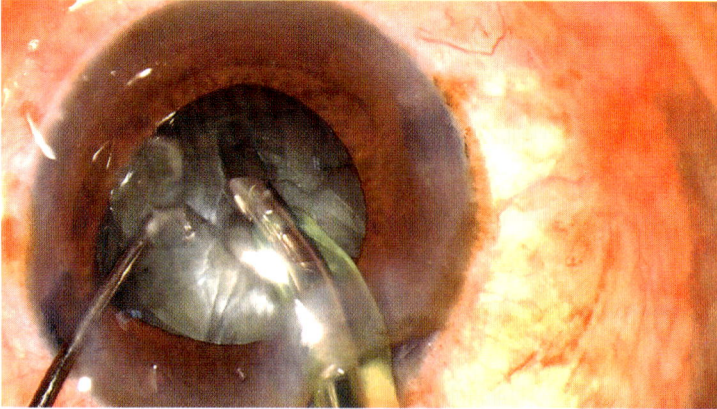

Fig. 1

Result

Hold is difficult.

Hold and Chop of Nucleus

Do's
- *Adequate or minimum energy is needed to engage the nucleus mass.*
- *Try to hold in the bulk of nucleus only.*

Observations (Figs. 2A and B)

- Hold is at posterior or deeper plane of nucleus.
- Debulking of nucleus mass seen at deeper plane.

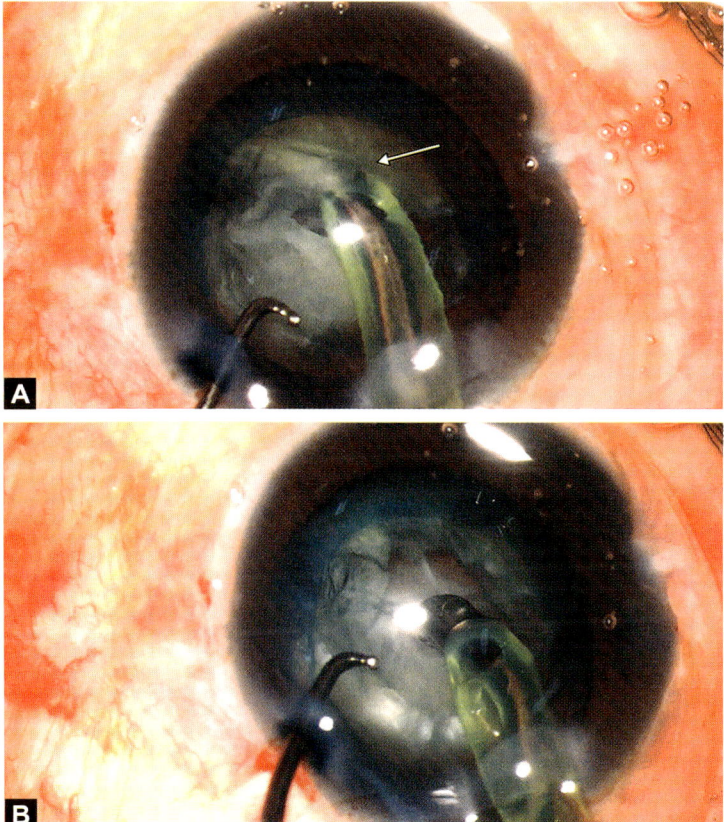

Figs. 2A and B

Result

There is a chance of posterior capsule rupture (PCR).

Do's
- *Hold should be in the middle bulky part of the nucleus.*
- *One should see engaged phaco tip at correct plane.*

Observation (Fig. 3)

Phaco tip is superficial to nuclear plane.

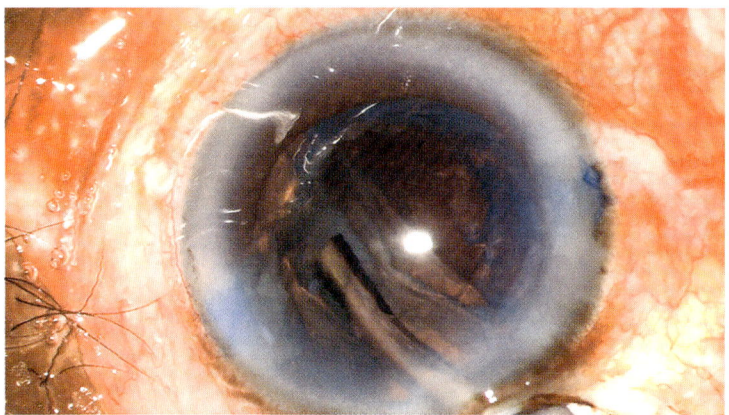

Fig. 3

Result

Unable to hold.

Do's
Phaco tip should be directed towards bulk of nucleus to hold.

Observation (Figs. 4A to D)

In all cases, phaco tip is placed at wrong position for hold.

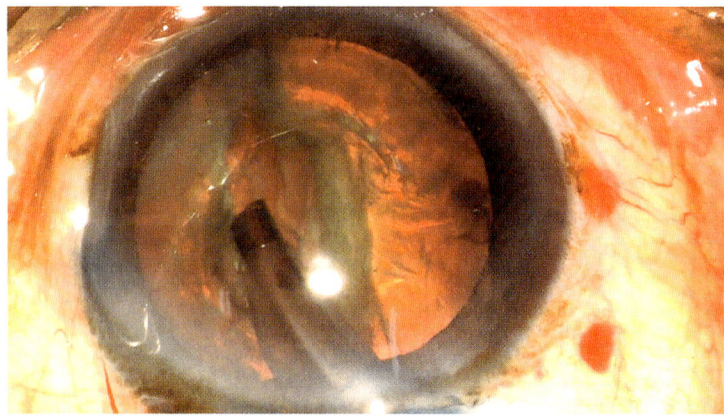

Fig. 4A

Hold and Chop of Nucleus

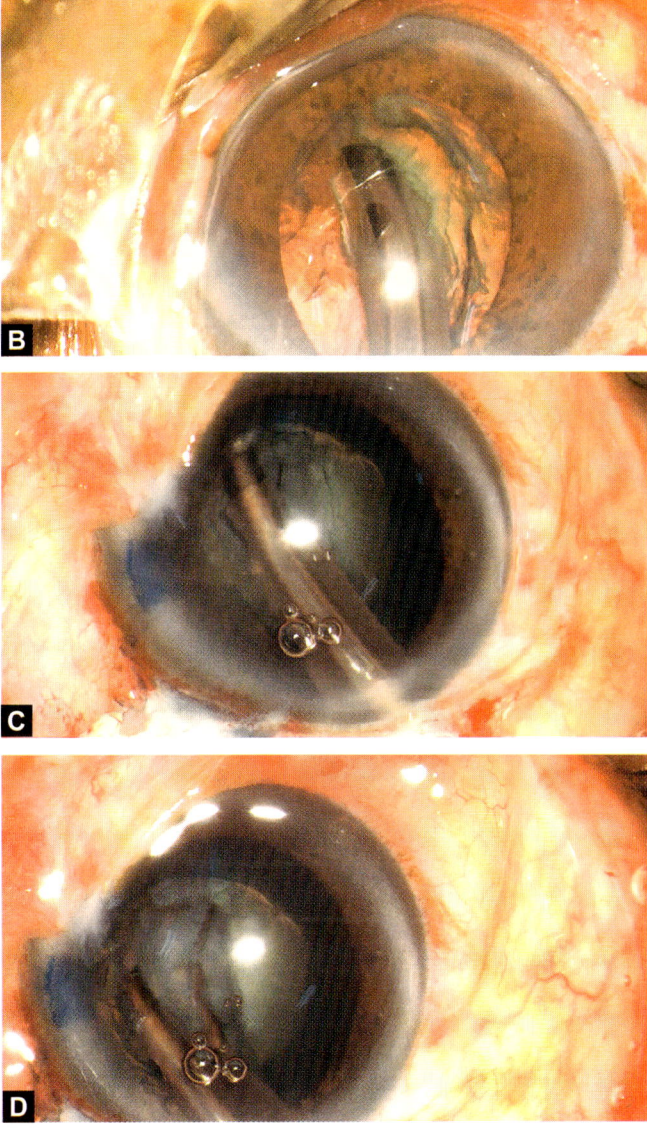

Figs. 4B to D

Result

Unable to hold.

> ### Do's
> - *Phaco tip should be always placed in the vicinity of nucleus.*
> - *Direction of the phaco tip should be toward the bulk of the mass or hard part of the nucleus.*

Observation (Figs. 5A and B)

Hold is near edge of nucleus.

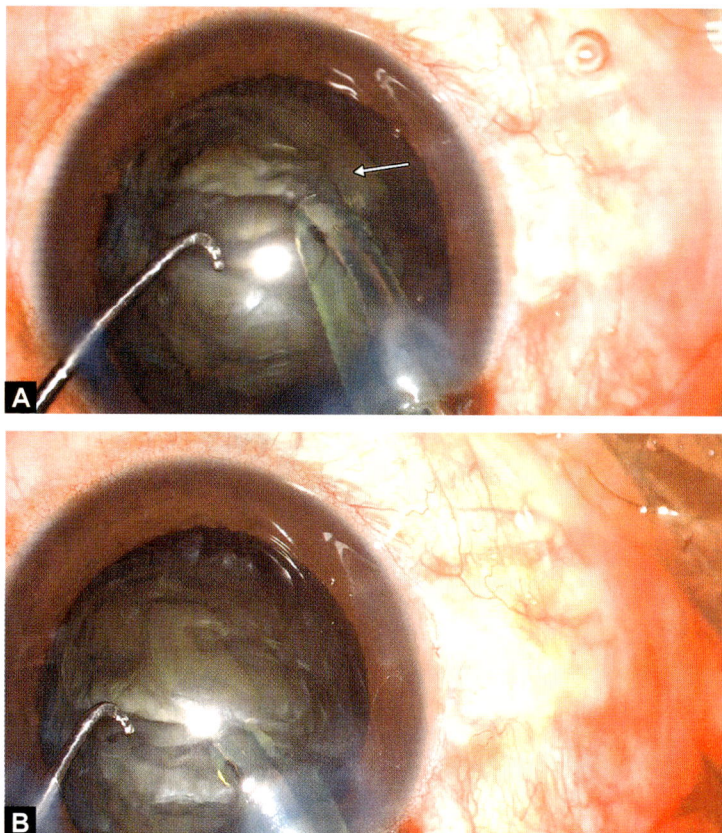

Figs. 5A and B

Result

Lifting of nucleus piece is difficult.

> *Do's*
> Hold should be done in center of nucleus.

Observations (Figs. 6A and B)

- Surgeon is attempting hold in wrong way.
- Energy used is more than needed in a wrong plane.

Hold and Chop of Nucleus

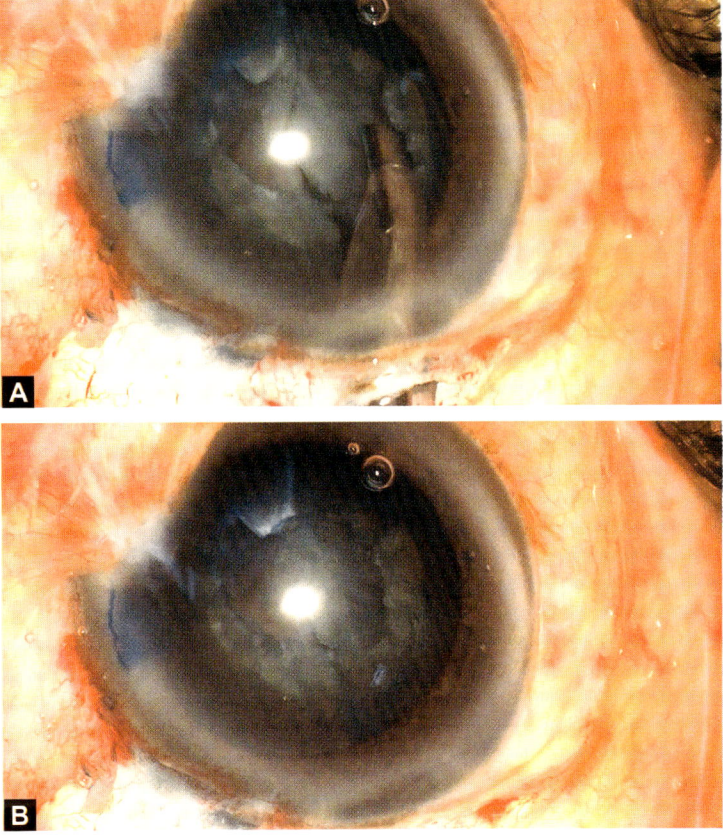

Figs. 6A and B

Results

- Surgeon fails to attempt hold.
- Bulk of nucleus mass is reduced.
- Bowl-like nucleus mass remains behind.

Do's
- *This may be a soft cataract.*
- *In a grade 2 cataract, this situation can occur, if energy used more than needed and phaco tip is angulated in wrong direction.*
- *Adequate parameters with better zero degree effect between phaco tip and nucleus mass are mandatory to hold in correct way to avoid this situation.*

Observation (Fig. 7)

Surgeon is pushing the piece of nucleus to engage during hold.

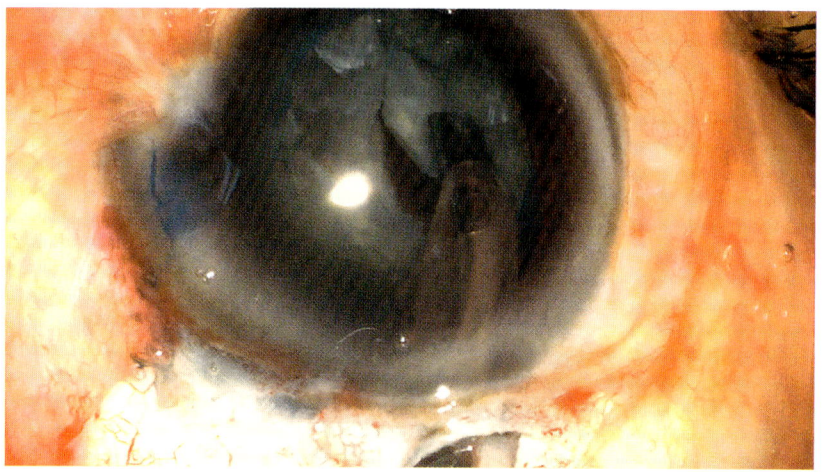

Fig. 7

Results

- Push effect may unable to hold.
- Pressure on zonules can occur.

Do's
- Do not push nucleus mass.
- Adequate vacuum and flow rate with minimum energy bring the piece toward phaco tip for hold.

PLACEMENT OF CHOPPER AND PHACO TIP IN HOLD AND CHOP

Observations (Figs. 8A to D)

- Half piece of nucleus pulled in the anterior chamber due to more vacuum and flow rate.
- Chopper is awkwardly put in the eye which is difficult to work.
- Crossing of chopper to phaco tip is noted.

Hold and Chop of Nucleus

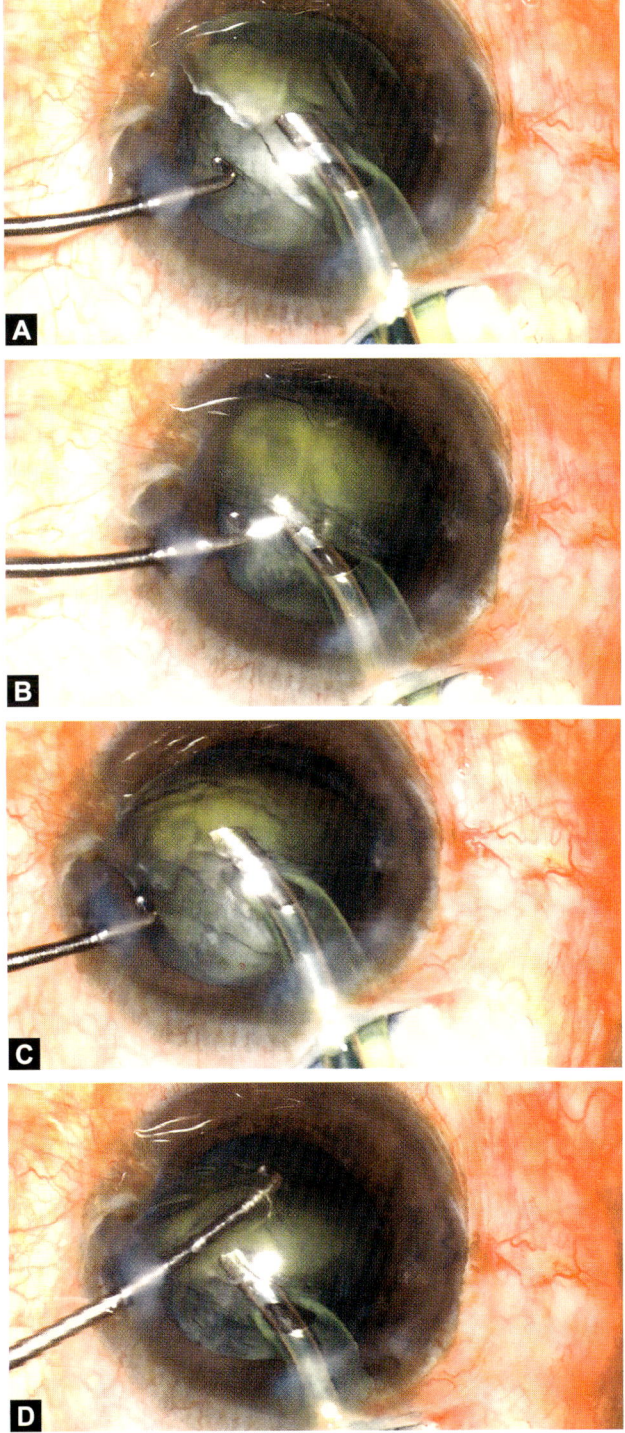

Figs. 8A to D

Results

- Hold and chop are difficult.
- Injury to cornea can occur.
- Due to awkward position of chopper, there is vertical stretching at incision site which may leak.

Do's
- Adequate vacuum and flow rate is needed to bring one edge of nucleus out of bag.
- Chopper should be always in horizontal position and point of chopper directed towards the main incision.
- Chopper should not cross phaco tip to avoid injury to cornea.

Observations (Fig. 9)

- Surgeon is trying to hold left side of mass superficially.
- Chopper is interfering with visualization.

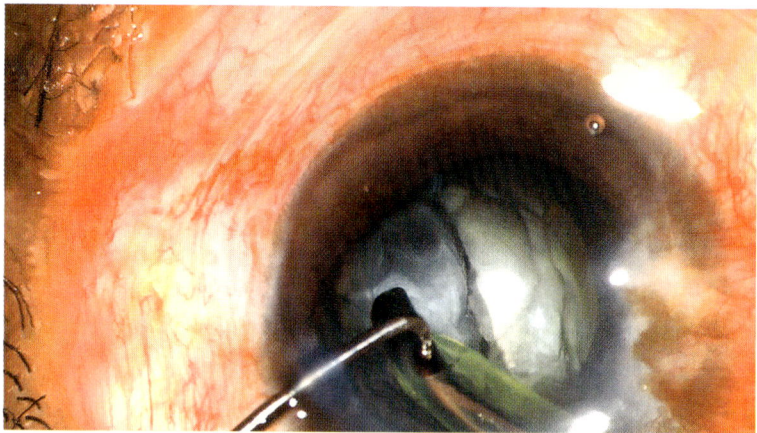

Fig. 9

Result

Due to superficial placement, bulk of the mass is reducing, which in further course, is difficult to hold.

Do's
- Location of hold should not be in the periphery.
- Hold should be near center as nucleus is more bulky there.
- Keep the chopper near the side port incision, which should not interfere with working of phaco tip (resting position of chopper).

Hold and Chop of Nucleus

Observation (Figs. 10A and B)

Surgeon is attempting to hold and chop near left side port incision.

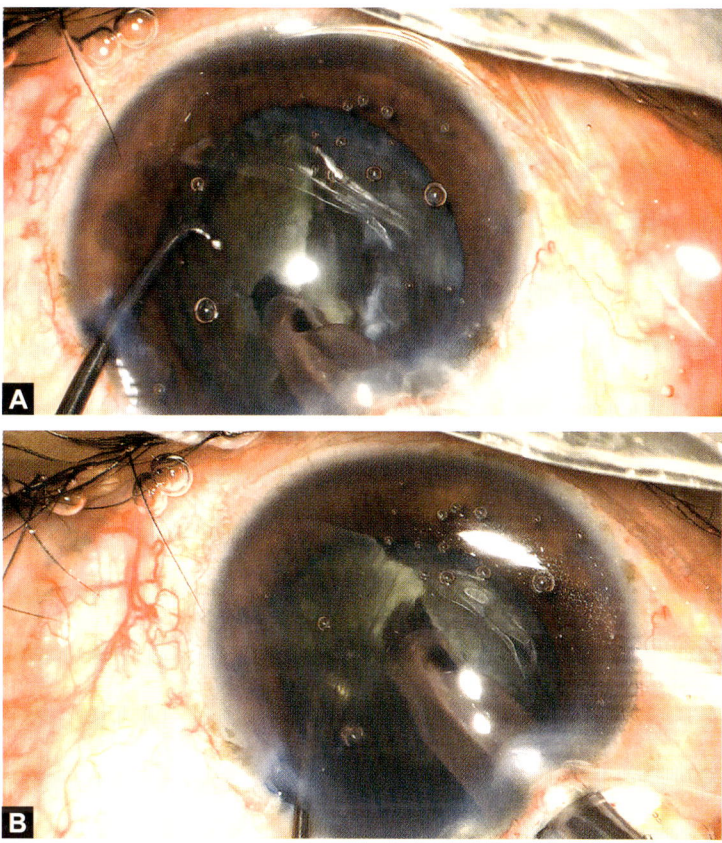

Figs. 10A and B

Result

Nucleus mass near side port is difficult to chop due to acute angulation of chopper.

Do's
Bring the nucleus mass to center for chop.

Observation (Fig. 11)

- Chopper crossed the phaco tip.
- Working plane of phaco tip and chopper is anteroposterior.

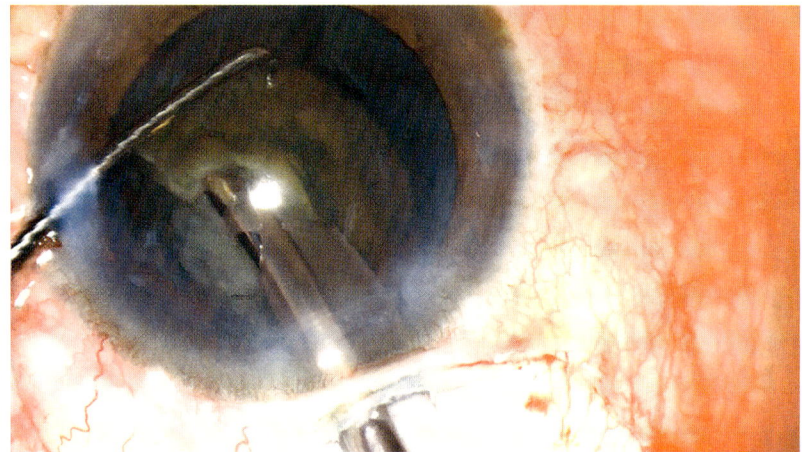

Fig. 11

Result

Chances of injury to cornea are more.

Do's
Do not cross chopper with respect to phaco tip.

Observation (Fig. 12)

Direction of chopper is parallel to nucleus mass during chop.

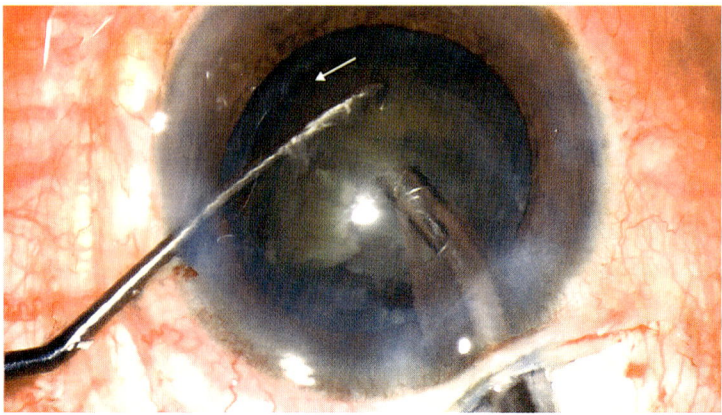

Fig. 12

Result

In this maneuver, hold can get dislodged due to direction of chopper.

> **Do's**
> Chopper should be perpendicular to long axis of nucleus mass.

Observation (Fig. 13)

Chopper is too periphery situated before chopping.

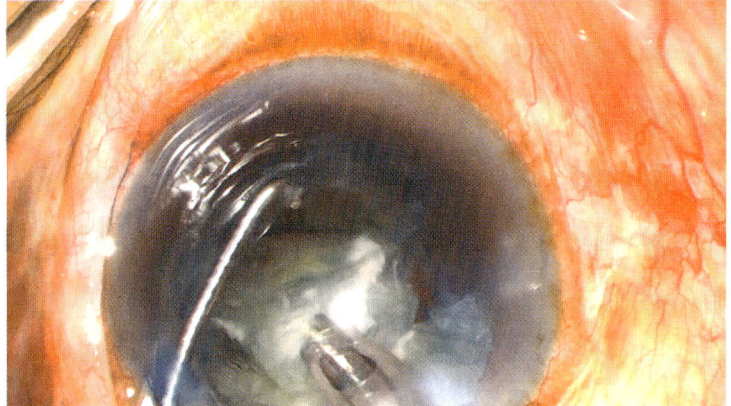

Fig. 13

Result

Injury to iris can occur.

> **Do's**
> - Chopping should be in the vicinity of phaco tip.
> - Edge of nucleus is seen which is an ideal point to start chopping.

Observations (Figs. 14A and B)

- Chopping started in periphery.
- Wrong direction and placement of chopper.

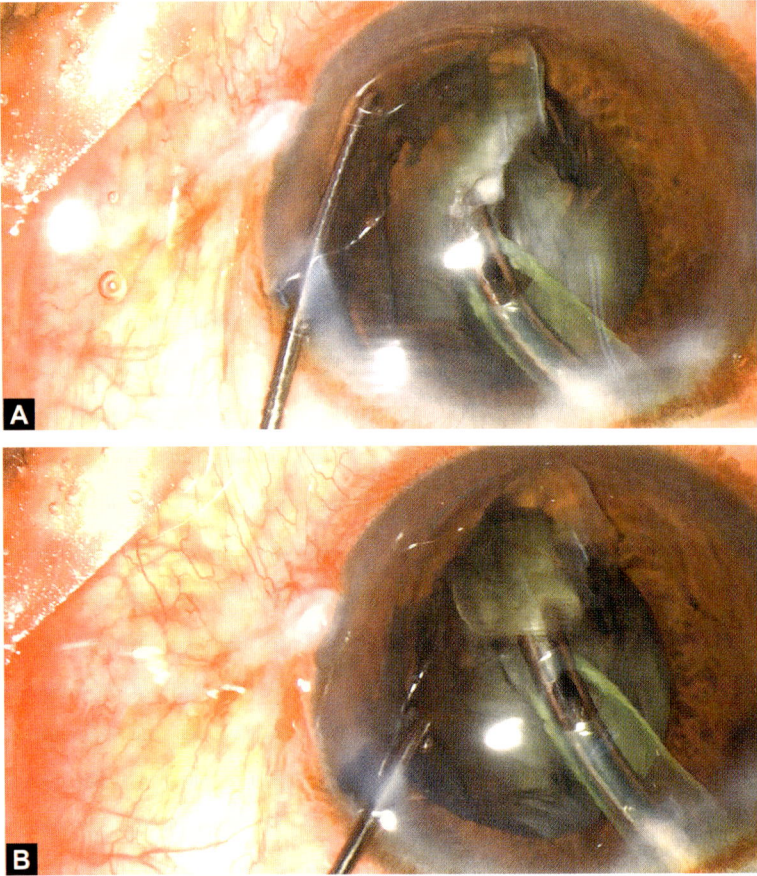

Figs. 14A and B

Result

Difficult to chop.

> ***Do's***
> - *Chopping should start at round edge of nucleus.*
> - *Direction of chopper is parallel or near parallel to phaco tip.*

Observation (Figs. 15A to C)

Hitting of chopper to phaco tip.

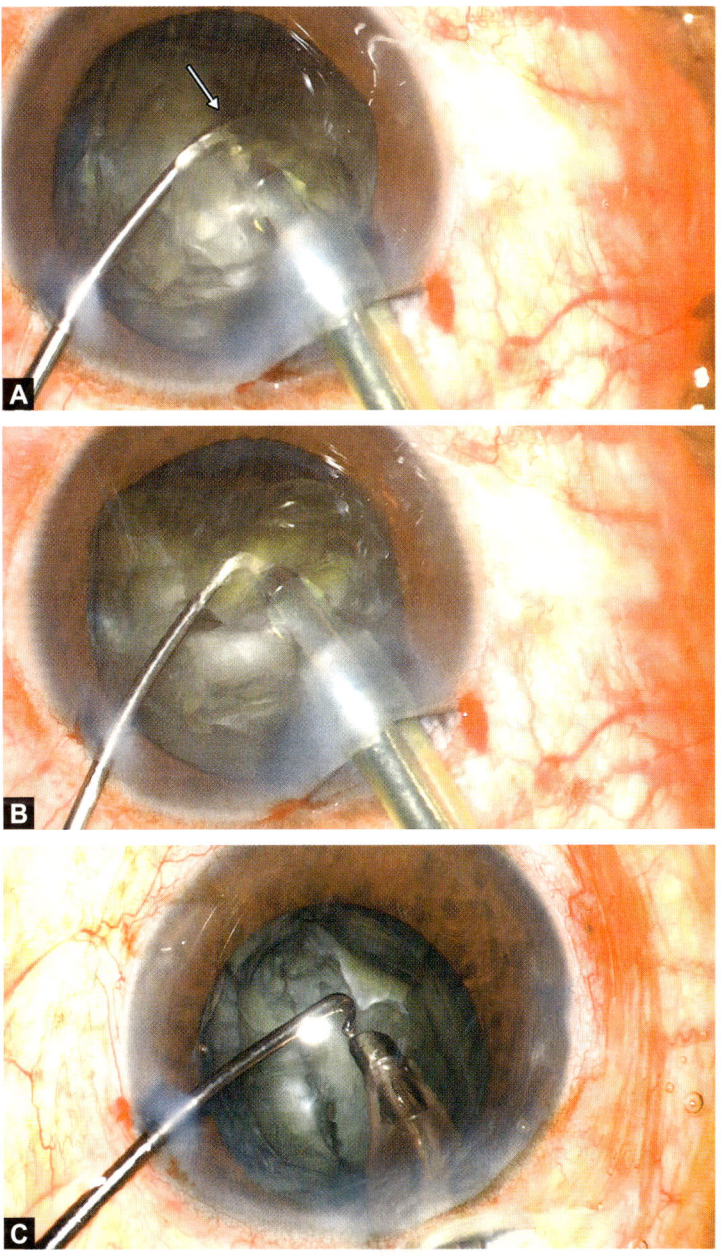

Figs. 15A to C

Result

Phaco tip can get blunt and damaged.

> **Do's**
> One should avoid touching of chopper to phaco tip.

Observations (Fig. 16)

- Phaco tip and chopper are not visible.
- Excessive pressure of chopper during chopping.

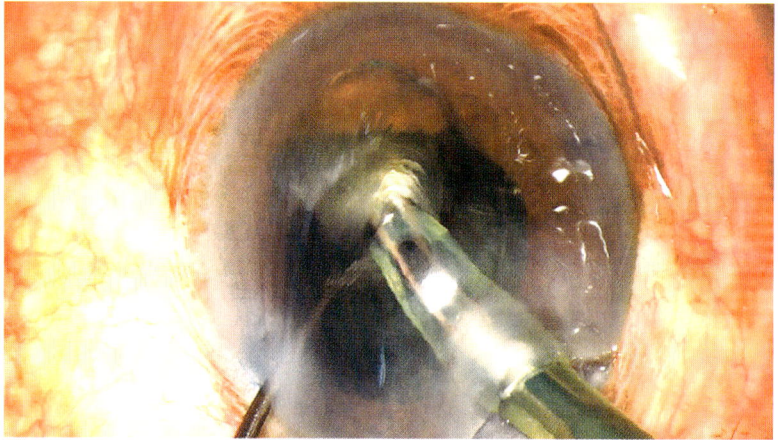

Fig. 16

Result

Chopper is placed posterior to phaco tip which can lead to PCR.

> **Do's**
> - Avoid pressure of chopper during chopping.
> - No need to chop small piece of nucleus.

Observations (Fig. 17)

- Hold is at apex.
- Placement of chopper behind the mass and directed towards phaco tip.

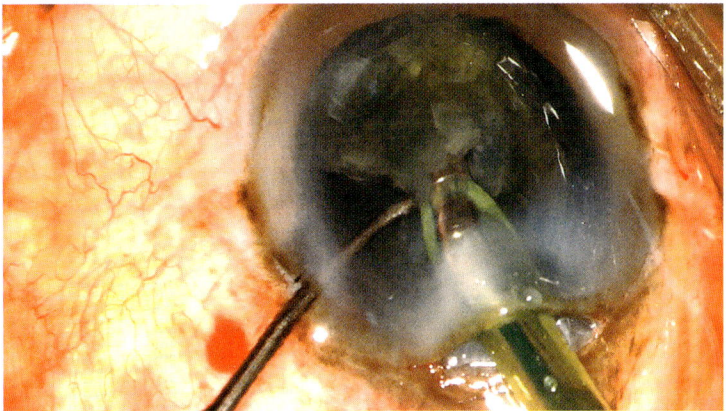

Fig. 17

Result

Chopper can damage phaco tip or sleeve.

Do's
Chopper should be placed from anterior aspect of nuclear mass to chop.

Observation (Figs. 18A and B)

Chopper is blindly gone behind piece.

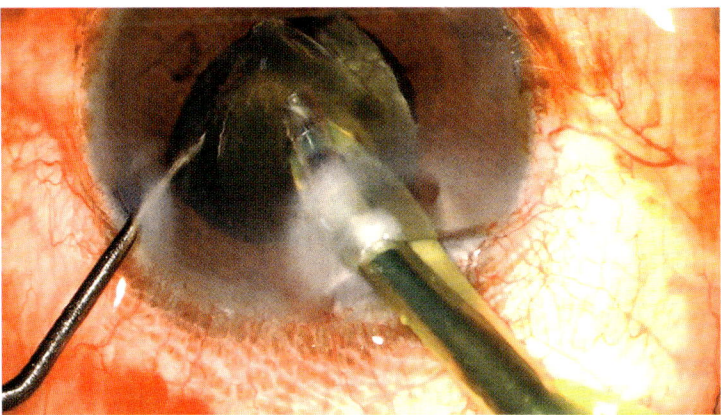

Figs. 18A

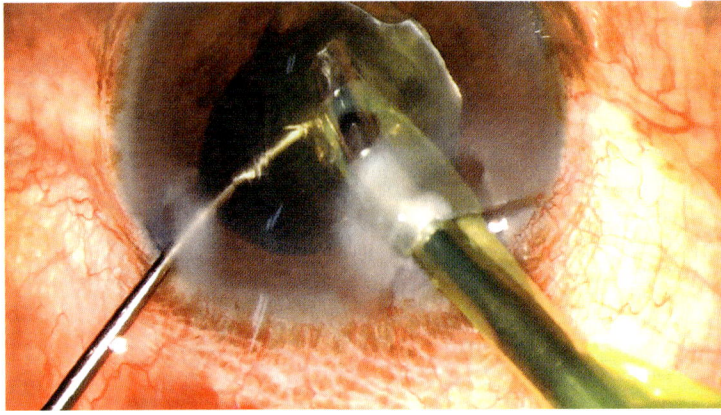

Fig. 18B

Results

- Chopping is difficult as hold is from round surface of the nucleus.
- Sleeve can get damaged.

Do's
- *Orientation of nucleus mass is not good for chop.*
- *Chopper should always be visible during chopping; otherwise PCR can occur.*

CASE SERIES OF HOLD AND CHOP

Observation (Figs. 19A to F and 20A to D)

Pulling of nucleus mass during hold.

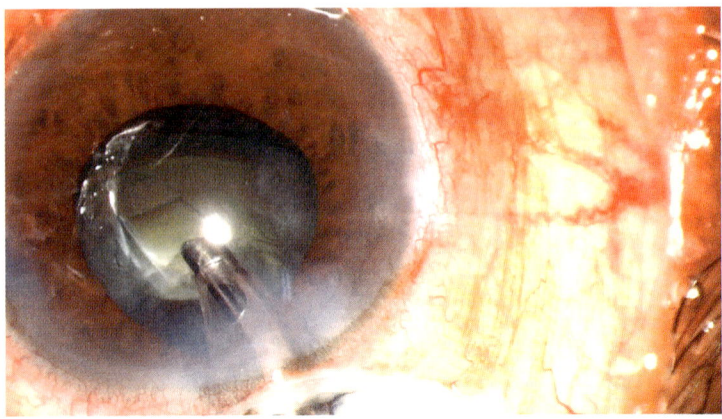

Fig. 19A

Hold and Chop of Nucleus 115

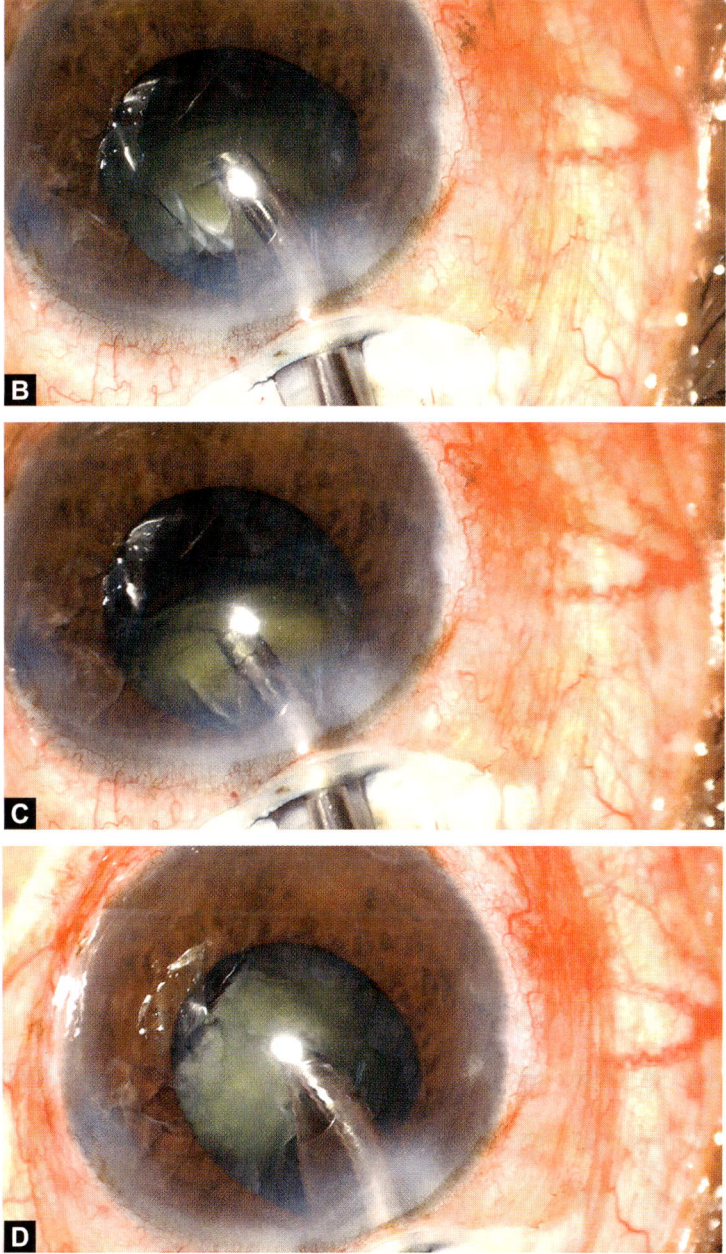

Figs. 19B to D

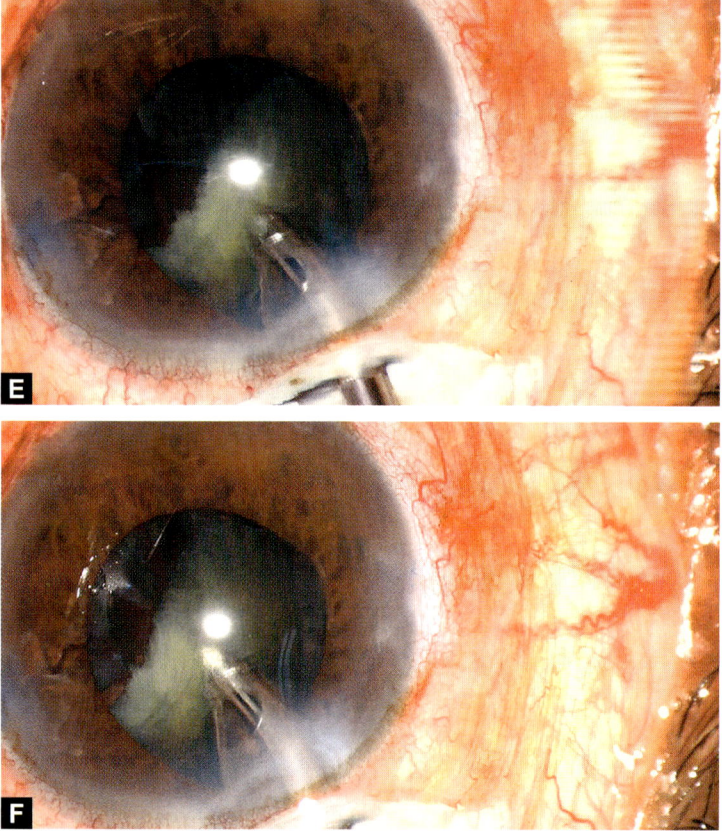

Figs. 19E and F

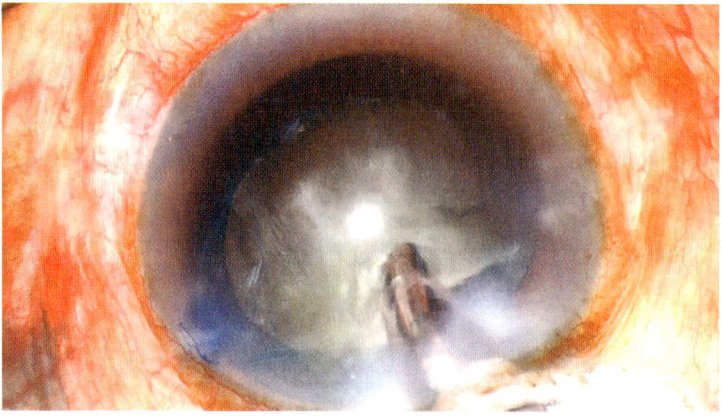

Fig. 20A

Hold and Chop of Nucleus 117

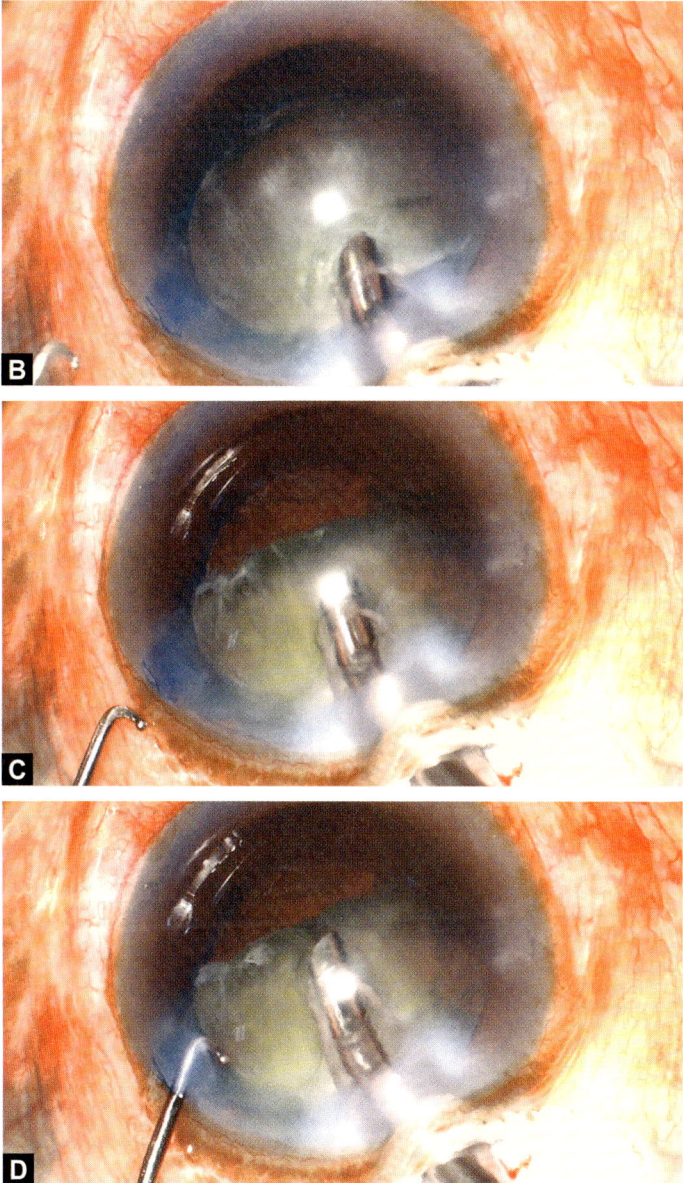

Figs. 20B to D

Result

Round mass of nucleus near the phaco tip is difficult to hold and chop.

Do's
- This situation is due to use of more vacuum and flow rate than needed and superficial placement of phaco tip.
- Adequate vaccum and flow rate with placement of phaco tip near the vicinity of mass is important to hold.

HOLD AND CHOP - DIFFERENT SITUATIONS (FIGS. 21A TO D)

Observations
- Surgeon is attempting hold and chop near the side port incision.
- There is no good space for chop.

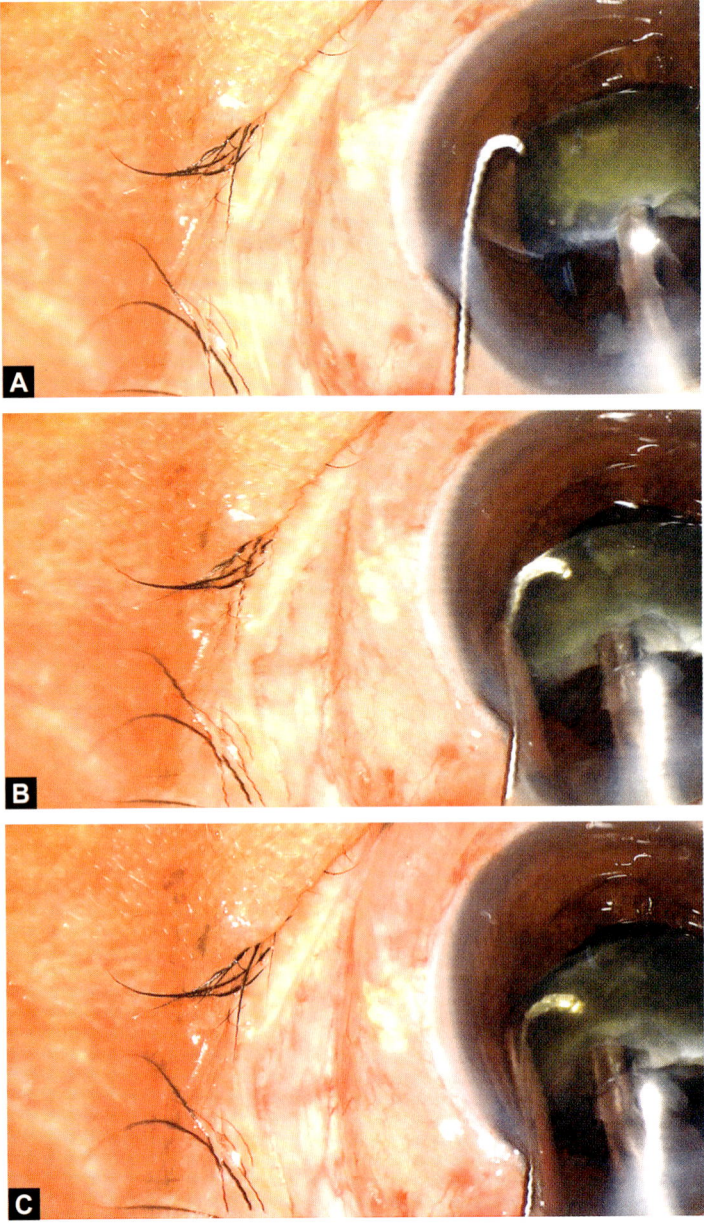

Figs. 21A to C

Hold and Chop of Nucleus

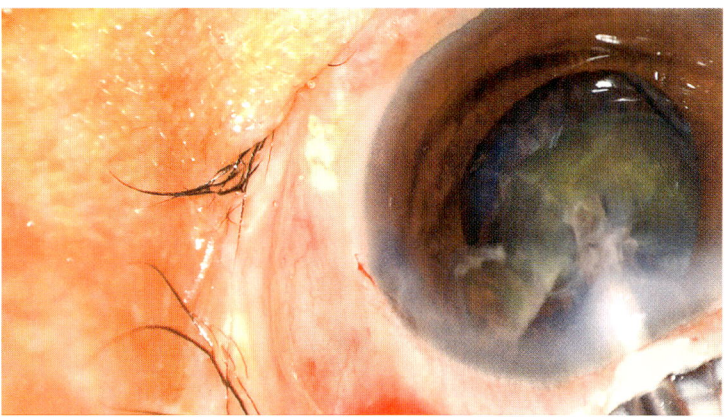

Fig. 21D

Results

- Acute angulation of chopper may be difficult to chop.
- Eyeball is distorted due to more pressure of chopper.

> ### Do's
> - Chopping should be done in the central safe zone.
> - One should not bring the mass of nucleus toward side port incision to avoid pressure and acute angulation of chopper.
> - Free movement of chopper is always helpful to chop the nucleus mass.

Observation (Fig. 22)

Hold is not in proper plane of nucleus.

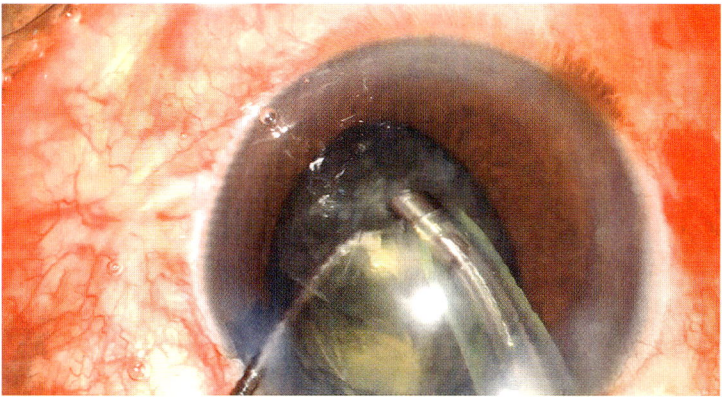

Fig. 22

Result

Chopping is not effective.

Do's
This bulk of nucleus can be emulsify directly without chop as it is not very bulky.

Observation (Fig. 23)

Piece of nucleus is parallel to phaco tip.

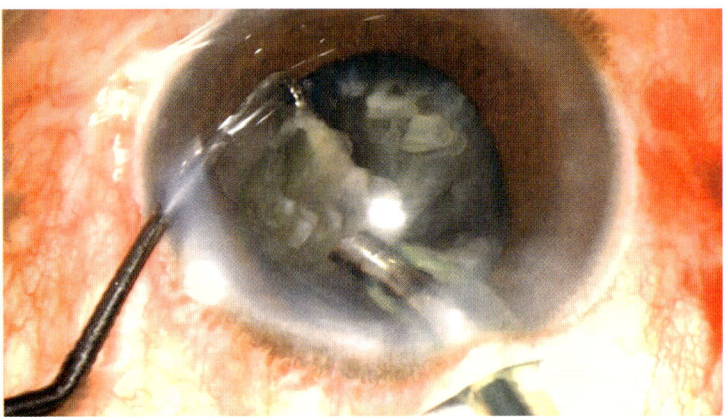

Fig. 23

Result

Chopping is difficult.

Do's
- *Plane of the nucleus and phaco tip should be perpendicular to each other.*
- *Chopping will be easy after proper alignment of nucleus.*

Observations (Fig. 24)
- Nucleus piece and phaco probe is not in one plane.
- Round surface of the nucleus faced toward phaco tip due to sudden increase in the vacuum and flow rate.

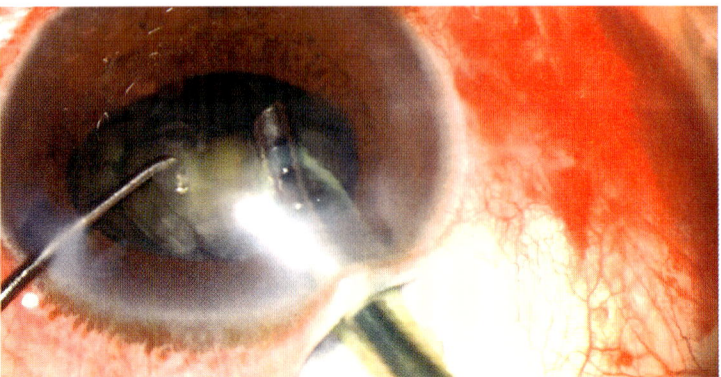

Fig. 24

Result

Bevel-down position of phaco tip may rupture posterior capsule.

> ### Do's
> - *Hold should be with adequate vacuum and flow rate.*
> - *Nucleus and phaco tip should be in one plane.*
> - *Phaco tip should be buried in the mass of nucleus which means that it should not be exposed before chop.*
> - *Chopper can push the piece forward and simultaneously phaco tip should go backward for proper alignment which results in better hold and chop.*

Observation (Fig. 25)

Big mass of nucleus is pulled toward incision.

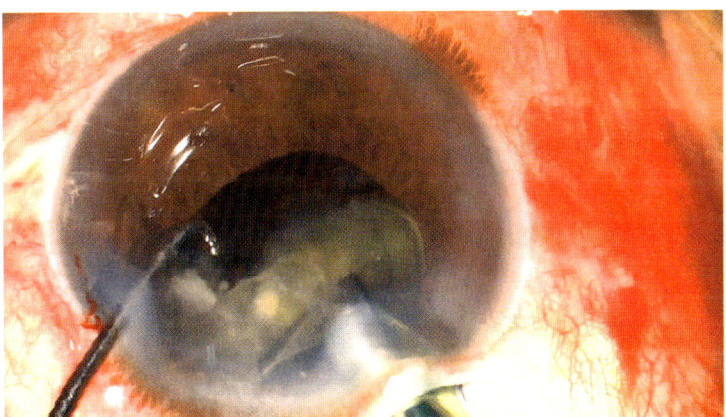

Fig. 25

Result

Chopping is difficult due to awkward position of chopper with respect to nucleus mass.

> ### Do's
> - *Hold and chop should be done generally in the center or near center.*
> - *This step should be in a slow manner to avoid such type of pulling.*
> - *Do not attempt to hold toward round surface of nucleus.*
> - *Perfect alignment of the nucleus piece needed for better hold and chop by pushing the nucleus back to center by chopper or phaco tip.*

Observations (Fig. 26)

- Chopper is hitting to the cornea.
- Anterior chamber is uneven.

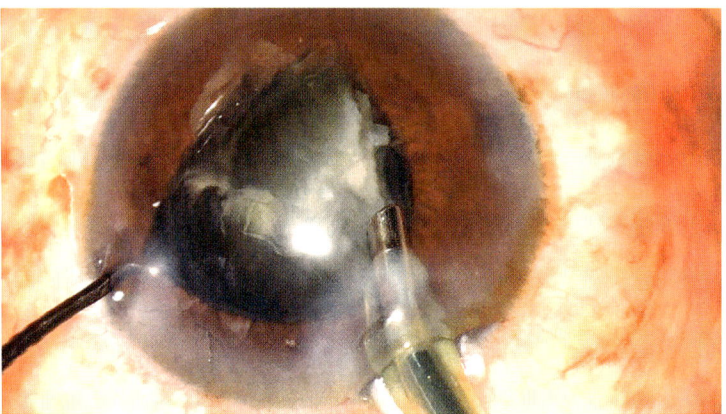

Fig. 26

Result

Injury to cornea or iris can occur due to chopper, phaco tip, and nucleus mass.

Do's
- *Placement of chopper should be horizontal to avoid injury to capsule, iris, and cornea.*
- *Phaco tip should not be near the incision site to avoid leakage and shallow anterior chamber.*

Observations (Figs. 27A and B)

- Surgeon is trying to chop small piece of nucleus.
- It is not an ideal placement of nucleus for chop.

Hold and Chop of Nucleus

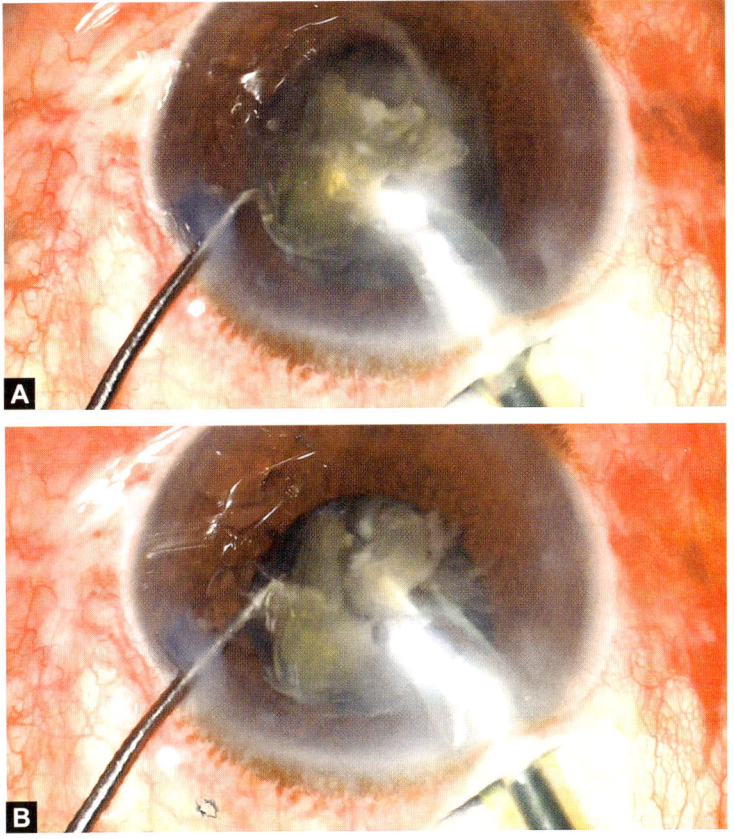

Figs. 27A and B

Result

Small piece of nucleus is difficult to chop.

Do's
No need to chop small piece of nucleus.

Observations (Figs. 28A and B)
- Nucleus mass is superoinferiorly placed.
- Inferior nucleus mass is oriented in reverse way, i.e. apex is seen.

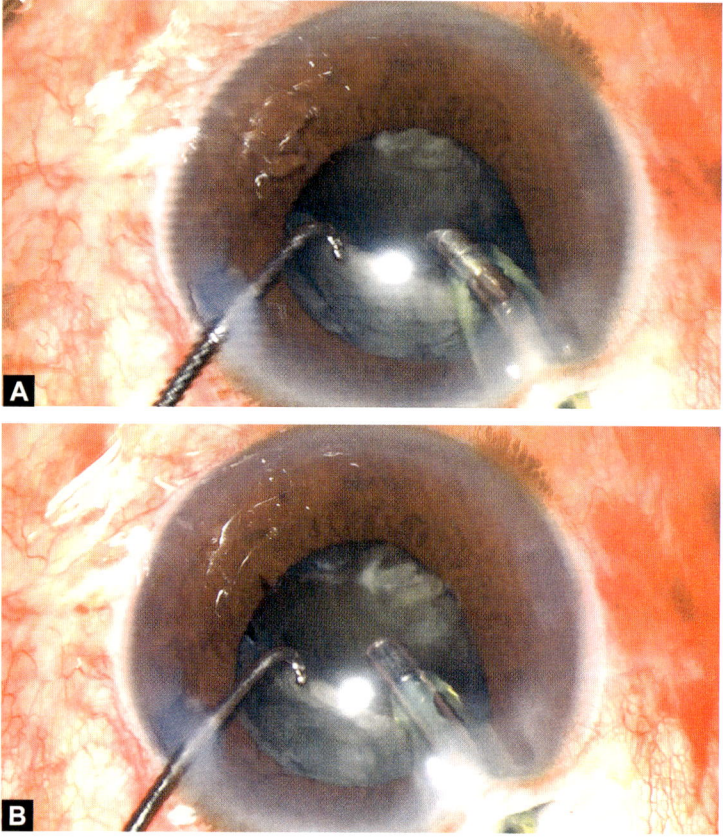

Figs. 28A and B

Result

This piece is difficult to chop.

> **Do's**
> Hold and chop is possible and easy once orientation of piece of nucleus in normal anatomical position.

Observations (Figs. 29A to C)

- Mass of nucleus is pulled near incision (Fig. 29A).
- Nucleus mass pushed toward center for chop (Fig. 29B).
- Placement of chopper is away from phaco tip (Fig. 29C).

Hold and Chop of Nucleus

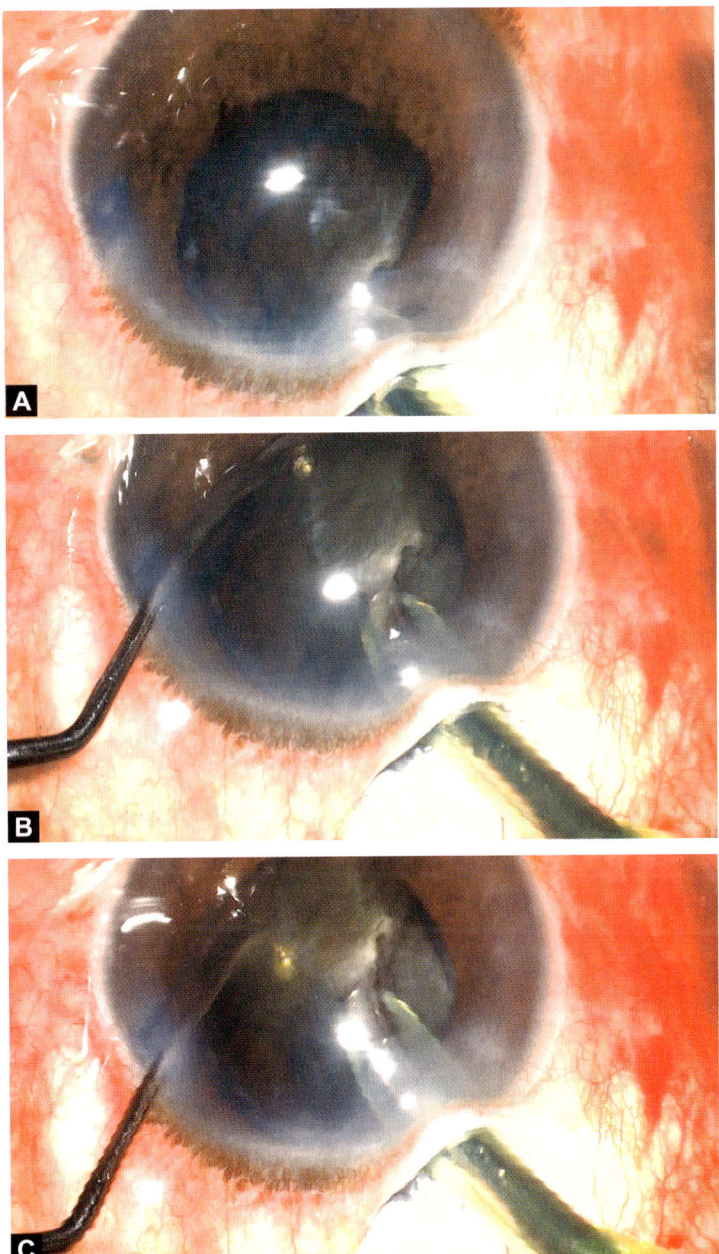

Figs. 29A to C

Result

Big mass of nucleus near incision can injure cornea.

Do's
- Do not pull nucleus mass toward incision which may injure cornea.
- Working of chopper should be near the phaco tip.

Observations (Figs. 30A to C)

- Nucleus is placed horizontally which is touching iris from both edges.
- Distortion of pupil.

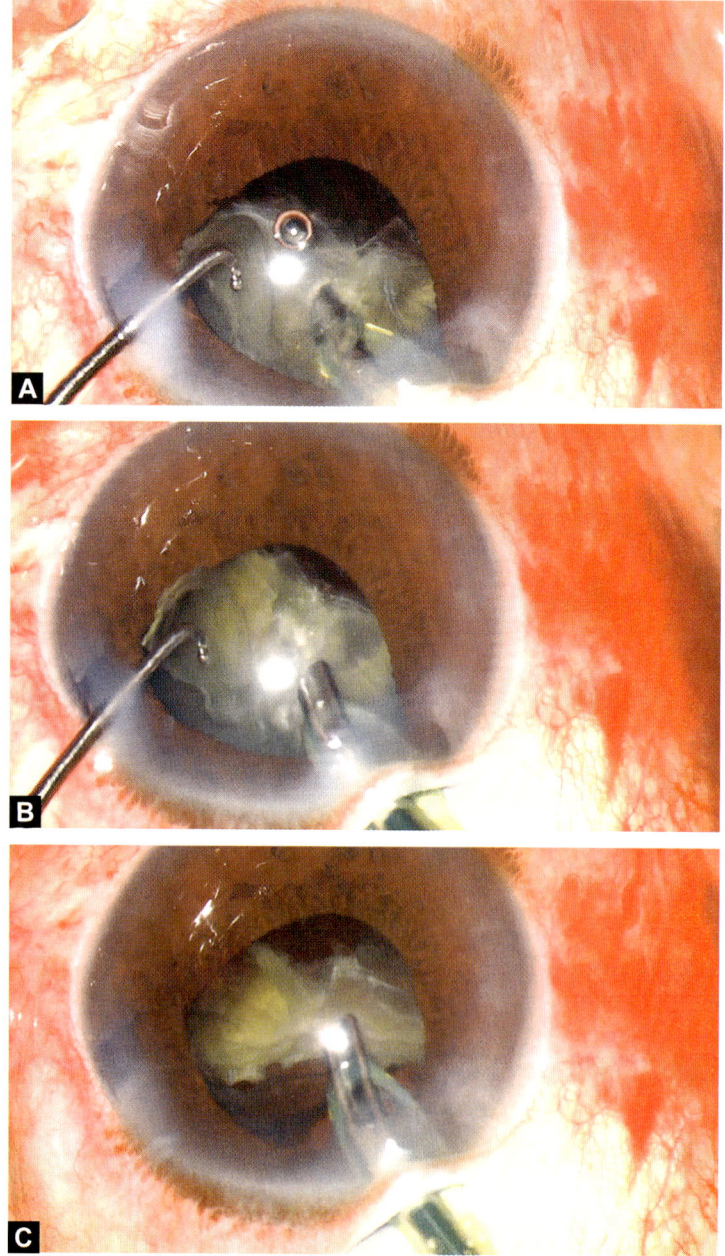

Figs. 30A to C

Result

Hold and chop is risky as big mass is situated in the bag.

> **Do's**
> Lift one edge of nucleus out of capsular bag for chop and further management.

Observation (Fig. 31)

Direction of phaco tip and chopper is not proper for hold and chop.

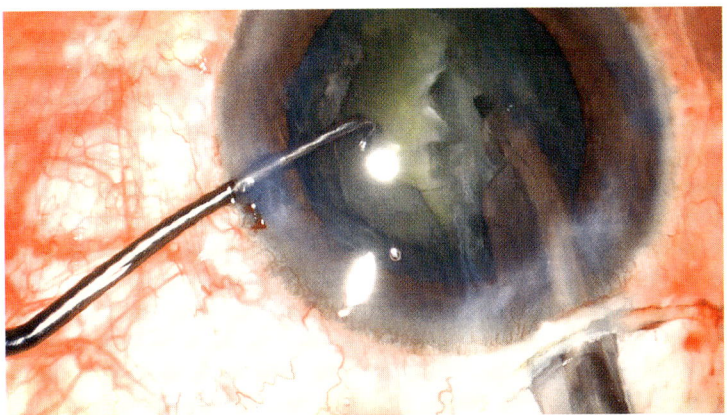

Fig. 31

Result

Surgeon has failed to attempt hold.

> **Do's**
> - Direction of the phaco tip should have zero degree effect with nucleus mass.
> - Chopper should be placed horizontal and kept ready for chopping once hold occurs.

Observation (Figs. 32A and B)

Phaco tip and chopper is not placed properly.

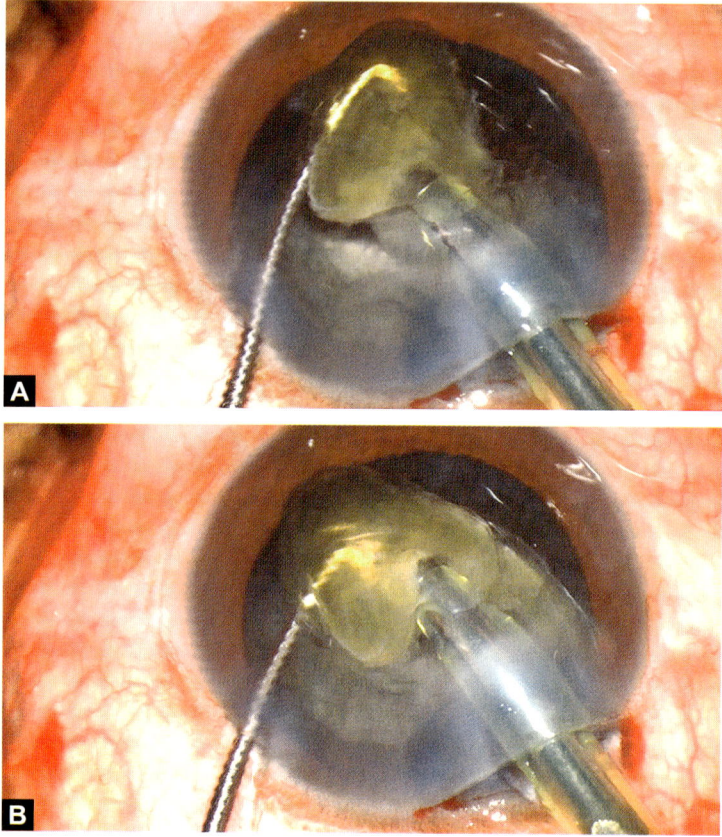

Figs. 32A and B

Result

Surgeon has failed to chop this piece.

> **Do's**
> - Direction of chopper should be 90° to longitudinal axis of the piece.
> - Due to wrong direction of chopper hold gets lost and rotation of nucleus mass can occur.

Hold and Chop of Nucleus

Observation (Figs. 33A to D)

Chopper is working blindly.

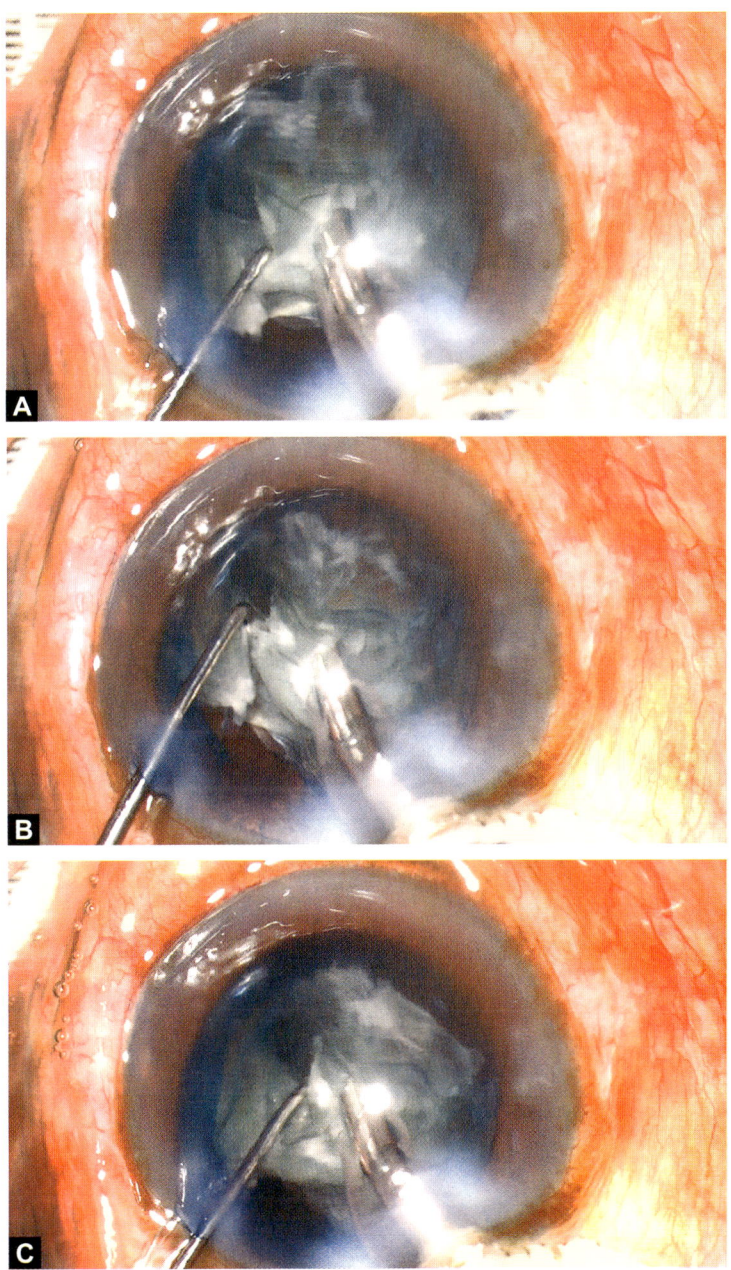

Figs. 33A to C

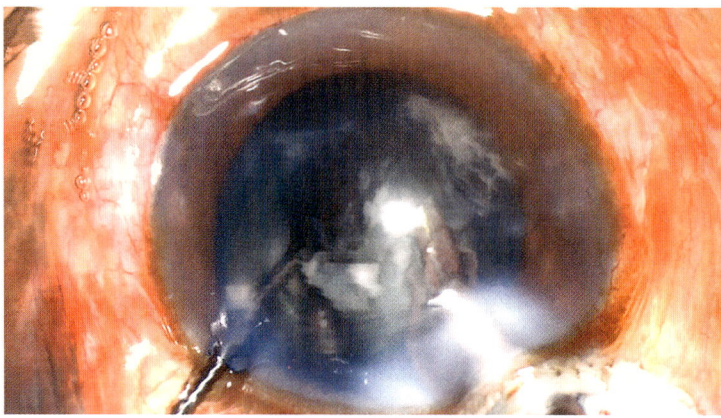

Fig. 33D

Result

Posterior capsule rapture can occur.

Do's
Phaco tip and chopper should be placed in one plane.

Observation (Fig. 34)

Shadows of drape disturb the view.

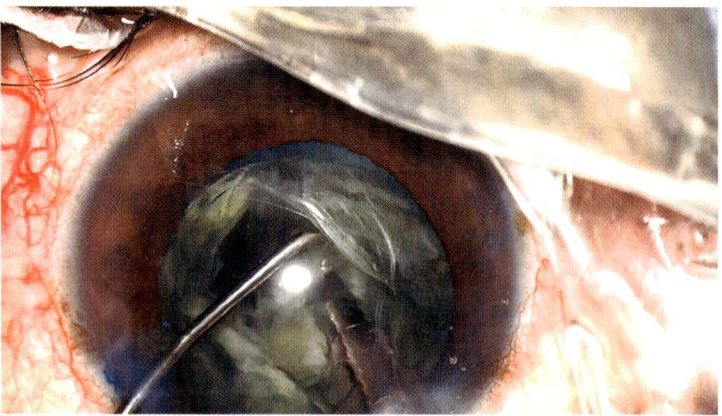

Fig. 34

Result

Visualization is difficult.

Do's
Putting a drape before surgery is an art.

CHAPTER 7

Removal of Pieces of Nucleus

INTRODUCTION

- This step is important in the sense that complications like hazy cornea, iris injury, and posterior capsule rupture are quite common during removal of small pieces.
- Knowledge of phaco fluidics is a must to do this step.
- Position of eye ball is also a considerable factor.
- Aspiration flow rate, vacuum, and energy are working together for effective removal of small pieces.

REMOVAL OF PIECES OF NUCLEUS

Observations (Fig. 1)

- Phaco tip is not visible.
- Chopper is pointed downward.

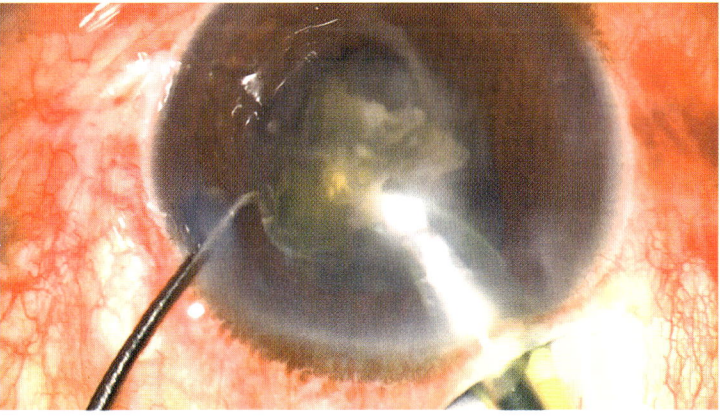

Fig. 1

Result

Chopper can damage iris or anterior capsule.

Do's

- *Phaco tip should be always visible during removal of piece.*
- *Placement of the chopper should be horizontal or oblique.*

Observation (Figs. 2A and B)

Phaco tip is over nucleus plane.

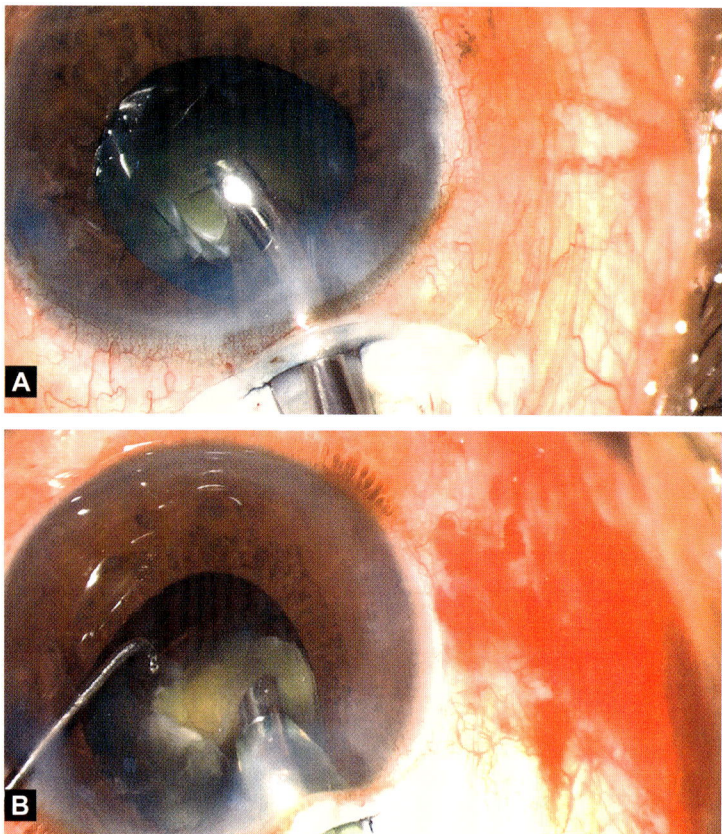

Figs. 2A and B

Result

Cornea can get hazy.

Do's

- *Nuclear piece and phaco tip should be in one plane.*
- *One can take help of chopper to bring nuclear piece and phaco tip in one plane.*

Observations (Fig. 3)

- Phaco tip is anterior to nucleus mass.
- Phaco tip directed downward.

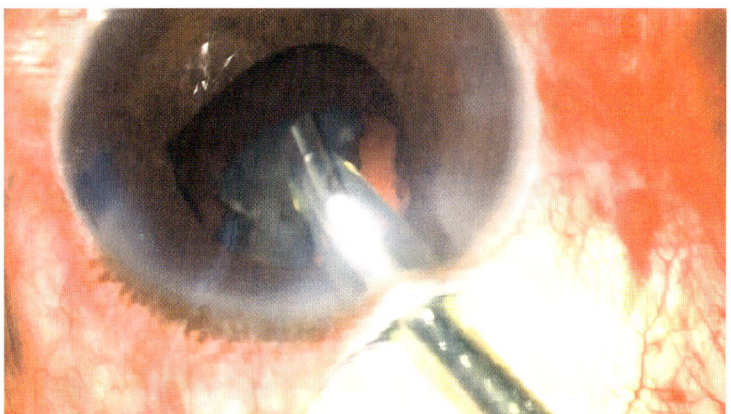

Fig. 3

Result

Chances of catching posterior capsule are more.

> **Do's**
> - *During removal of piece, Kelman tip should be usually bevel sideway position.*
> - *Bring the phaco tip from center to toward incision for better followability for easy removal of piece.*
> - *Alignment of nucleus piece with respect to phaco tip is better, once phaco tip moves back toward incision.*

Observations (Fig. 4)

- Phaco tip is anterior to nuclear mass.
- Eating is in the soft part of nucleus.

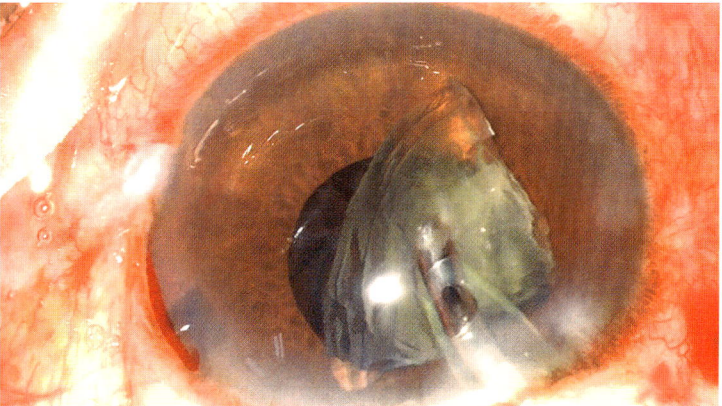

Fig. 4

Result

Cornea can get hazy.

> **Do's**
> - Reorient the piece in such a way that both phaco tip and mass should be in one plane and start emulsifying from apex of mass which is ideal way to deal with it.
> - In the same situation, use minimum energy which can be controlled with foot-pedal.

Observation (Fig. 5)

When surgeon is removing one piece, other piece is touching the cornea.

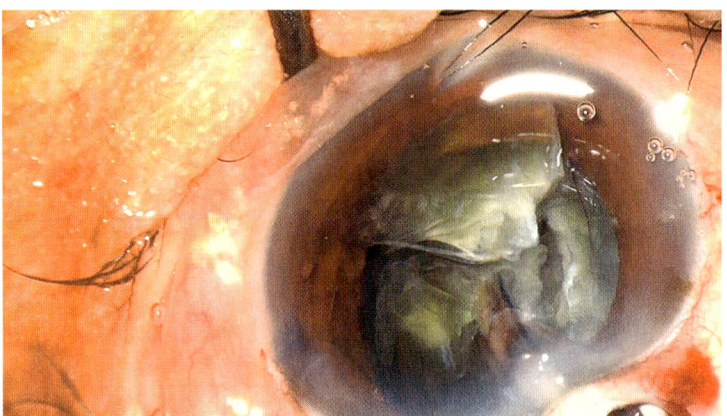

Fig. 5

Result

Cornea can get hazy due to rubbing of nucleus mass.

> **Do's**
> Try to remove nuclear piece which is moving in anterior chamber first to avoid damage to cornea.

Observation (Fig. 6)

Surgeon is trying to remove the piece which is in the bag.

Removal of Pieces of Nucleus

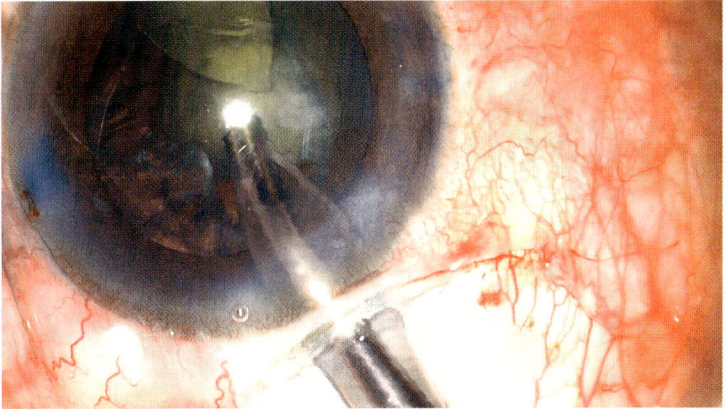

Fig. 6

Result

Chances of catching posterior capsule are on higher side.

Do's
- Surgeon should remove the piece which is in anterior chamber first.
- While emulsifying the piece in the bag, all parameters should be cut down.

Observations (Fig. 7)

- Direction of phaco tip is downward.
- Phaco tip is working without nuclear mass, i.e. in empty space.

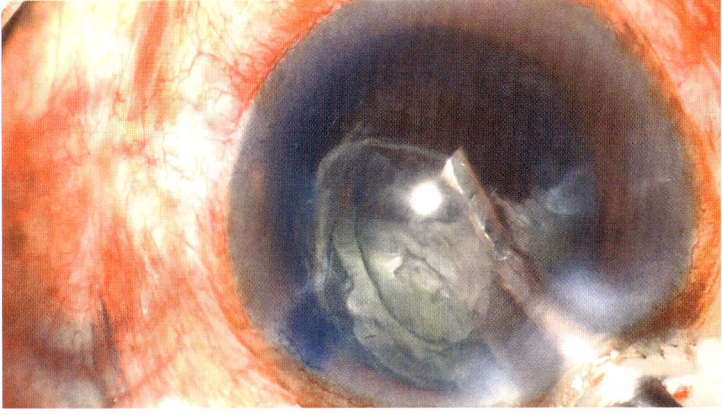

Fig. 7

Result

Posterior capsule rupture can occur.

> **Do's**
> - Phaco tip should be in plane of nucleus mass.
> - Bulk or mass of nucleus should be in front of phaco tip before eating.
> - Reorientation of bulky nuclear mass can be done with chopper for hold and chop or removal of pieces.

Observations (Fig. 8)

- Phaco tip is exposed.
- No mass is in front of the tip.

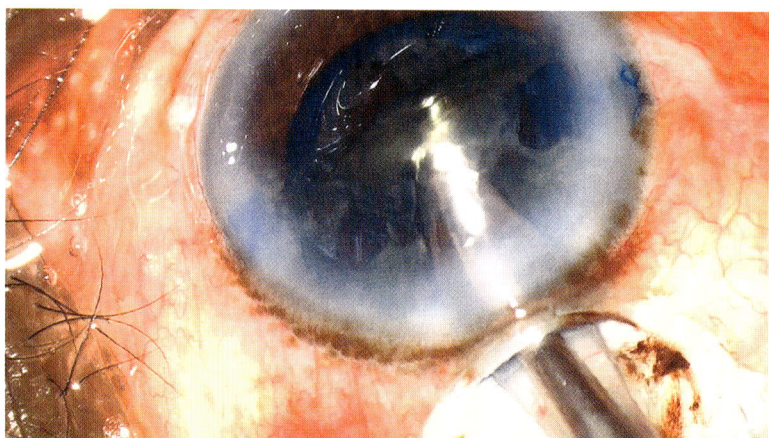

Fig. 8

Results

- Chances of catching iris and capsule are common.
- Exposed part of the tip can release energy to cornea which can get hazy.

> **Do's**
> Do the reorientation of piece in such a way that bulk of the mass with one edge of the nucleus or apex should be in front of the phaco tip for eating.

Observation (Fig. 9)

Triangular shape of pupil indicates uneven anterior chamber.

Removal of Pieces of Nucleus

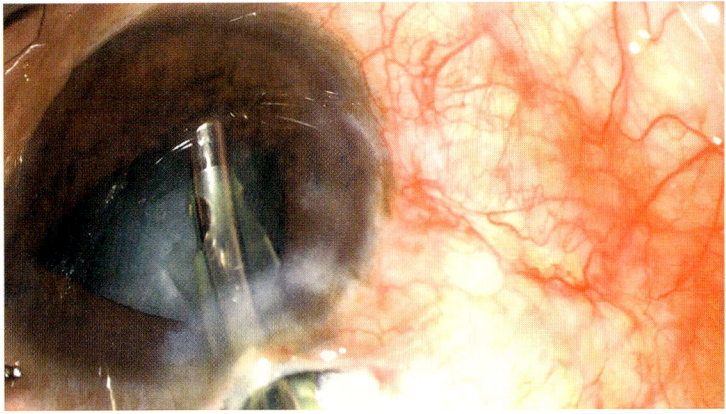

Fig. 9

Results

- Uneven anterior chamber hampers water current, better phaco fluidics, and followability of pieces toward phaco tip.
- Phaco tip may catch iris.

Do's
- *Phaco tip should be embedded in the bulk of nucleus and lift it out in the anterior chamber to settle the iris to make anterior chamber even.*
- *As iris is stucked at side port, other option to form anterior chamber is to bring out phaco tip and push viscoelastic from side port incision.*
- *Even and formed anterior chamber is important for better phaco fluidics.*

Observations (Fig. 10)
- Size of nucleus piece is big.
- Phaco tip is working in the center.

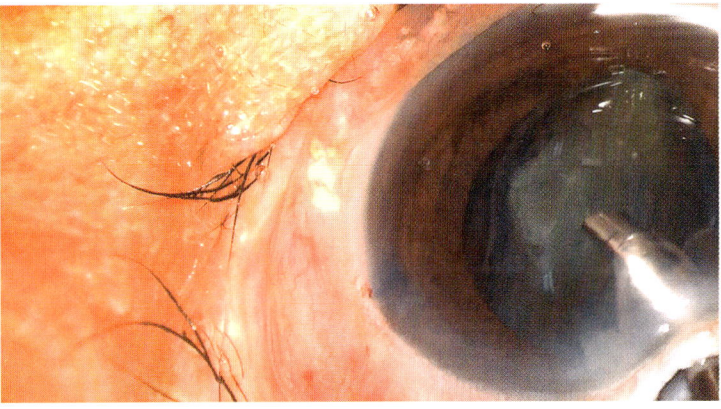

Fig. 10

Result

Orientation of piece is not good for eating.

> **Do's**
> - Try to reorient the piece first.
> - Next step is hold and chop.
> - Removal of chopped piece.
> - After reorientation, if surgeon is not comfortable to hold and chop then start emulsifying of piece from one edge of nucleus.

Observation (Fig. 11)

Orientation of nucleus piece is reversed (upside down).

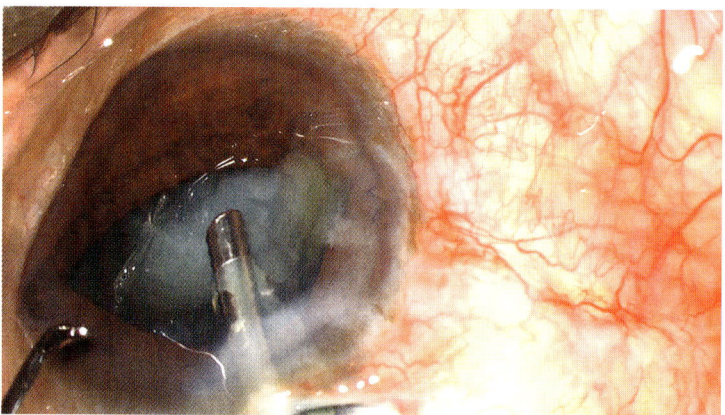

Fig. 11

Result

Difficult to eat the nucleus piece.

> **Do's**
> - Chopper should not be placed as iris is stuck to side port incision.
> - Pushing the nuclear piece down may settle the iris.
> - Try to reorient the nuclear piece, i.e. nucleus should be at its anatomical position before removal.

Observation (Fig. 12)

Eating of nucleus in the periphery.

Removal of Pieces of Nucleus

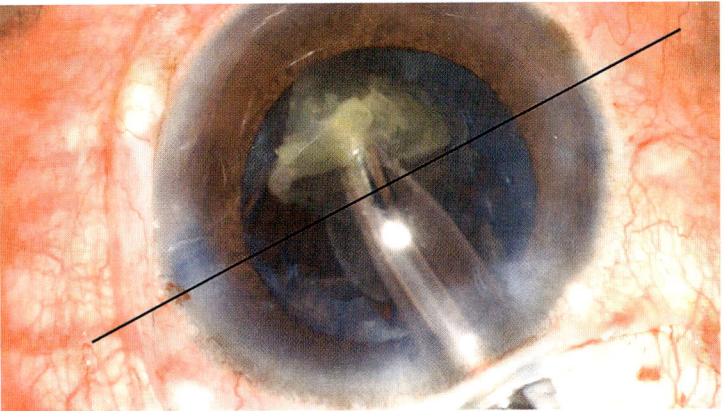

Fig. 12

Result

Injury to iris or capsule can occur.

Do's
- One should not emulsify the piece periphery to avoid injury to iris and capsule.
- One should not cross 180° to eat pieces.
- Phaco tip can move periphery to just hold and bring piece of nucleus toward center.

Observations (Fig. 13)
- Phaco tip is in the periphery.
- Visualization of the distal end of phaco tip is difficult.

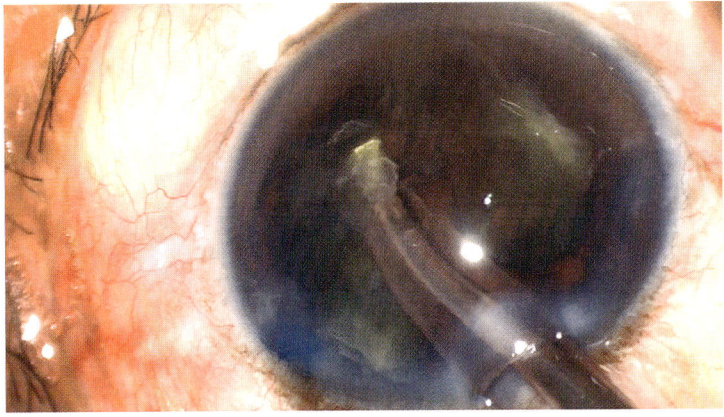

Fig. 13

Result

Injury to iris, zonular dialysis or posterior capsule rupture can occur.

> **Do's**
> - Eating of pieces should be in the center.
> - Phaco tip can go to periphery for just to hold the piece with adequate vacuum and flow rate to bring in the center.

Observations (Fig. 14)

- Eyeball is shifted to left side due to pressure of phaco tip on eye ball.
- Visualization is difficult.

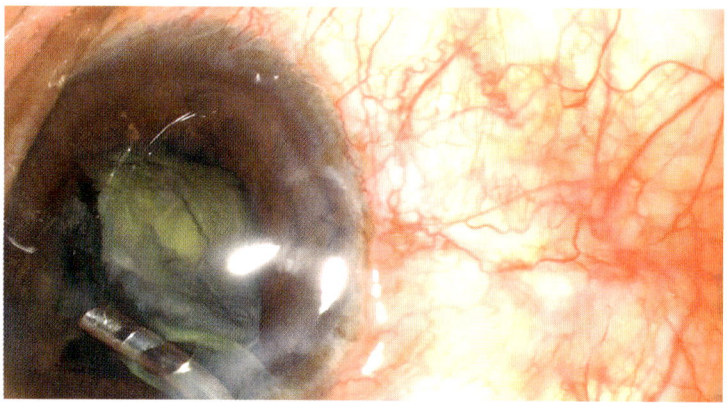

Fig. 14

Results

- Leakage of wound can occur.
- Anterior chamber is uneven.

> **Do's**
> Avoid the pressure on eyeball, as this position may hamper the phaco fluidics.

Observation (Fig. 15)

Angulation of chopper toward the nucleus is acute and awkward in position.

Removal of Pieces of Nucleus 141

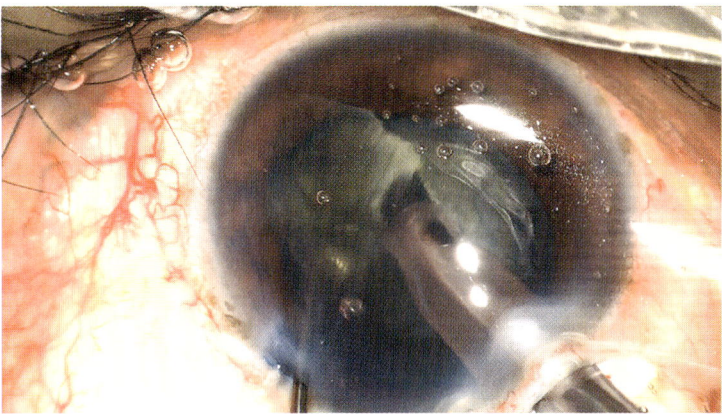

Fig. 15

Result

More pressure of chopper can leak the wound which interferes with better phaco fluidics.

Do's
- Avoid pressure of chopper.
- Take the chopper out to improve phaco fluidics and removal of pieces.

Observation (Fig. 16)

Touching of phaco tip to the chopper.

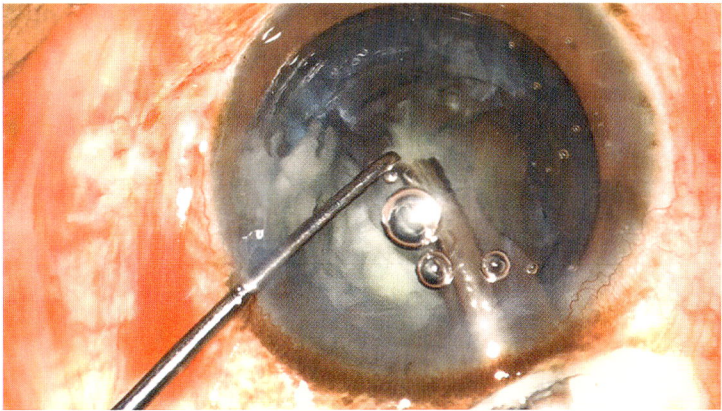

Fig. 16

Result

Phaco tip can get blunt.

> **Do's**
> - Avoid touching of phaco tip to chopper, otherwise tip can get damaged.
> - Placement of chopper should be horizontal or oblique.
> - Chopper should be placed near the side port incision to maintain the horizontal position of eyeball (Resting position).

Observations (Fig. 17)

- Surgeon is trying to remove big mass of nucleus.
- Both edges of the nucleus piece may hit iris from behind.

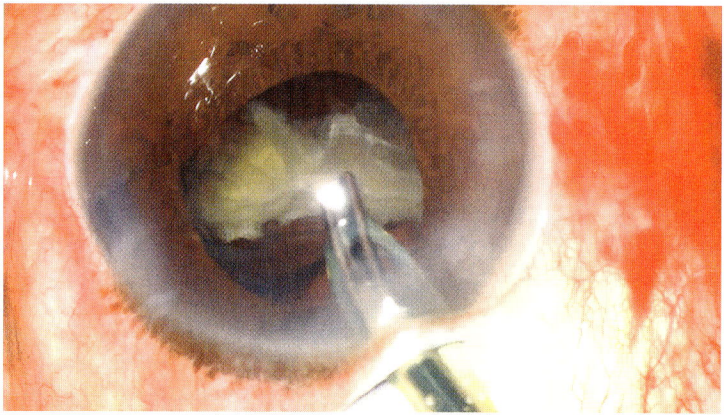

Fig. 17

Result

Pupil can constrict during surgery.

> **Do's**
> - Try to catch peripheral part of nucleus and lift it out of the bag and start emulsifying.
> - In this position, surgeon should do hold and chop.

Observations (Fig. 18)

- Iris is incarcerated in side port incision.
- Bulk of nucleus may press the iris from behind.

Removal of Pieces of Nucleus

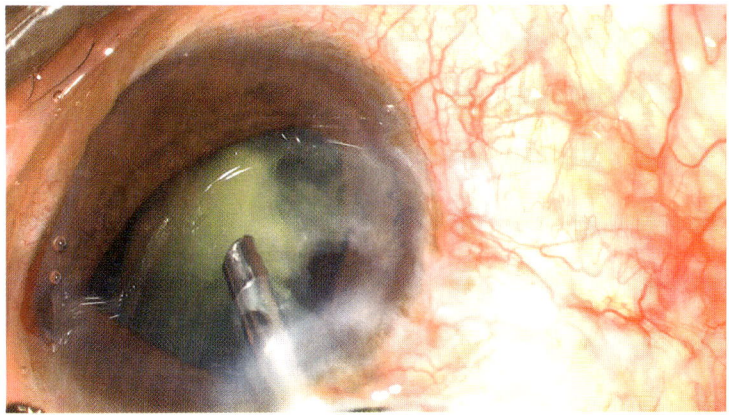

Fig. 18

Result

Iris injury can occur due to nucleus mass.

Do's
- Uneven anterior chamber is not a good prerequisite for removal of piece.
- We cannot put the chopper in the eye when iris is incarcerated in the side port incision so no hold and chop is advisable.
- At this situation, put the phaco tip quickly at the right side edge of the nucleus and with adequate vacuum and flow rate and try to emulsify the piece.

Observations (Fig. 19)
- Iris is stucked at side port.
- Uneven anterior chamber.

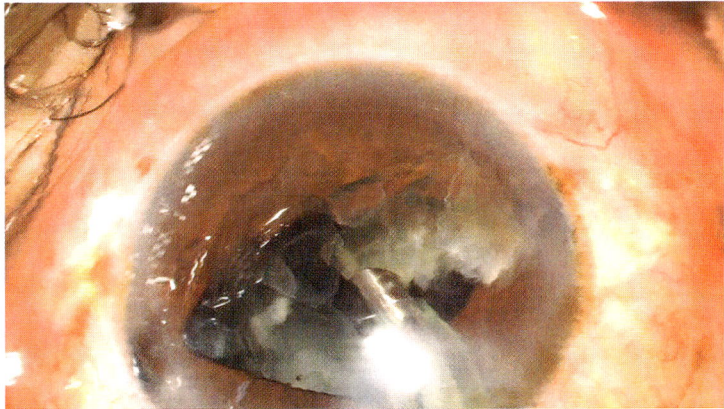

Fig. 19

Result

Phaco fluidics is not working.

> ### Do's
> - Due to uneven anterior chamber, phaco fluidics is not normal which may cause difficulty to remove pieces.
> - Removal of pieces with phaco tip without help of chopper is advisable.

CHAPTER 8

Irrigation - Aspiration of Epinucleus and Cortex

INTRODUCTION

- Irrigation-aspiration is an important step in the sense that this procedure is in empty bag, i.e. without hard part of lens.
- Most dreaded complication—posterior capsule rupture and zonular dialysis is quite common in this step.
- Both coaxial and bimanual irrigation-aspiration cannulas should be placed very gently in the capsular bag.
- To understand the principle and concept of this procedure is really important in practice.

IRRIGATION-ASPIRATION

Observation (Fig. 1)

Hitting of the iris with visco cannula.

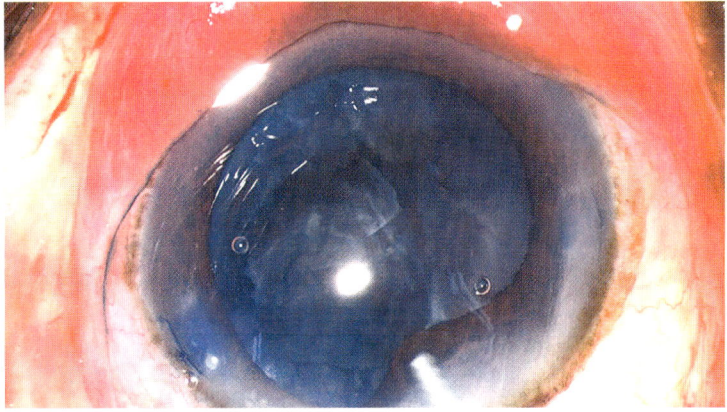

Fig. 1

Result

Constriction of pupil can occur.

Do's

- Shallow anterior chamber and wrong direction of the visco cannula is responsible to touch iris.
- Fill the anterior chamber first near incision then introduce visco cannula further in anterior chamber.
- Direction of the visco cannula should be parallel to iris.

Observation (Figs. 2A to C)

Putting viscoelastics, before irrigation-aspiration, may stretch the cortex and epinucleus.

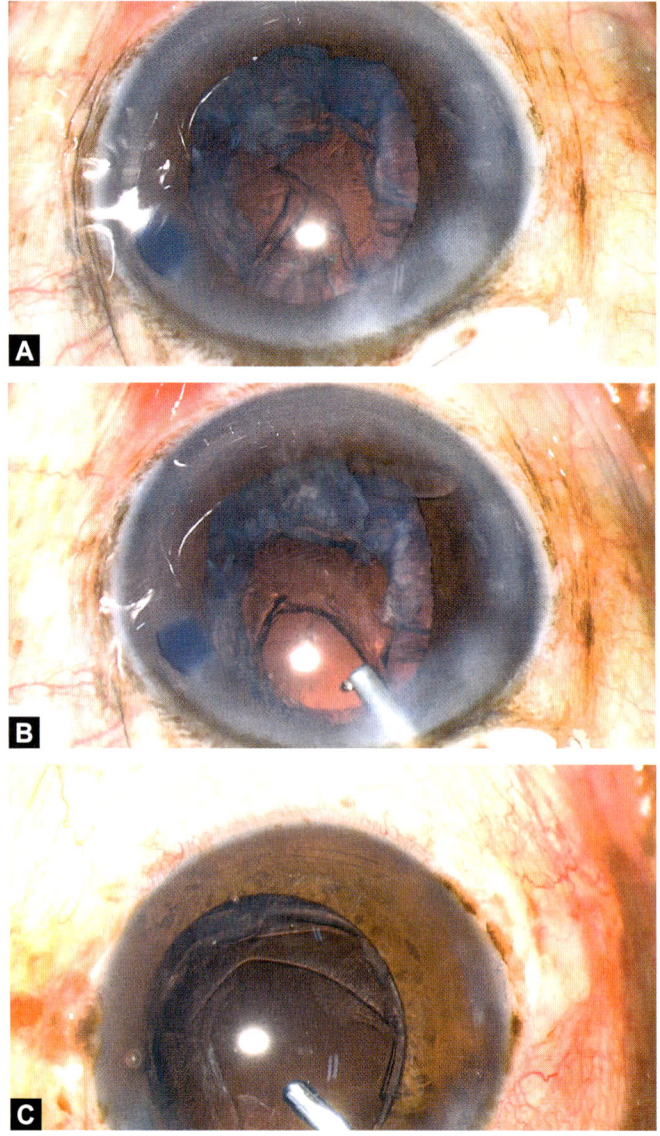

Figs. 2A to C

Result

Sometimes it looks like posterior capsule rupture (PCR).

> *Do's*
> - *Putting viscoelastics before start of irrigation-aspiration is an art.*
> - *Always fill anterior chamber first and then bag.*
> - *The cortex and epinucleus should be put back to its normal anatomical position which is easy for removal.*

Observation (Fig. 3)

Aspiration port of irrigation-aspiration cannula not seen due to air bubbles.

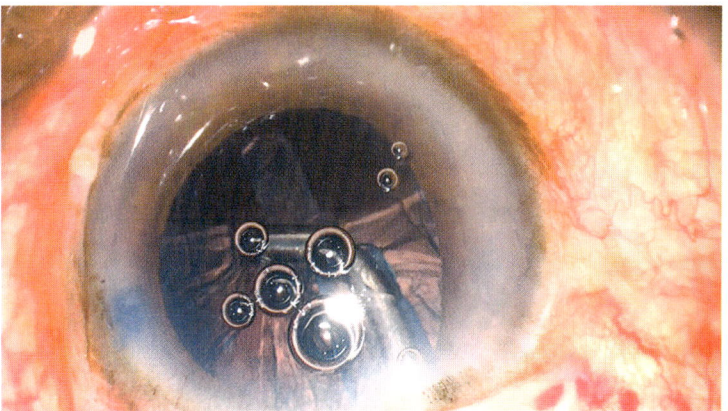

Fig. 3

Results

- Irrigation-aspiration is difficult.
- Visualization is hampered due to lot of air bubbles.

> *Do's*
> - *There should not be any air bubbles for better visualization before start of this step.*
> - *Subincisional cortex removal is always crucial so visual clarity of the field should be good.*

Observation (Figs. 4A and B)

Aspiration of viscoelastics only without soft tissue.

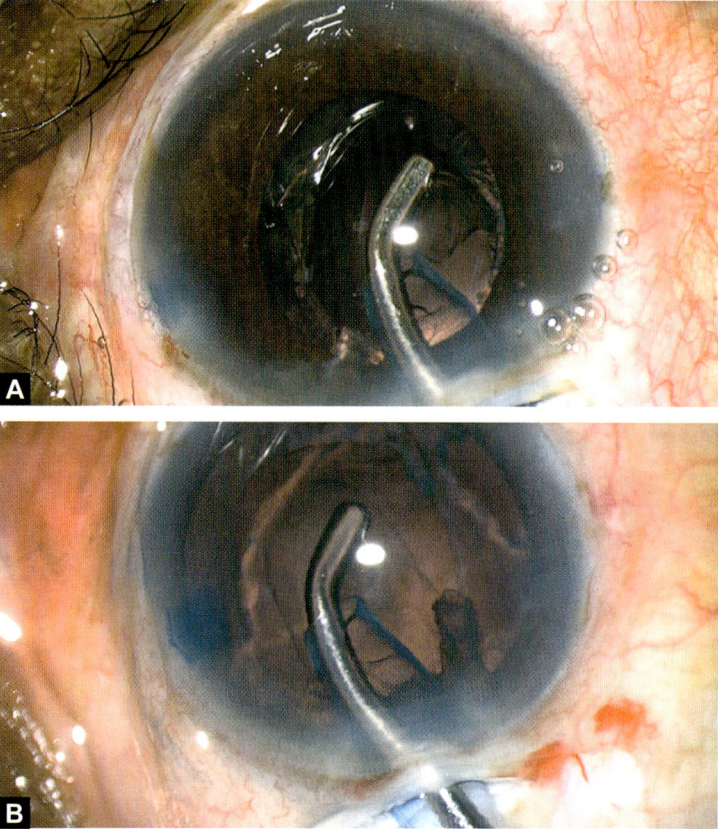

Figs. 4A and B

Result

Anterior chamber and bag may collapse.

> **Do's**
> Irrigation-aspiration cannula should be near the soft tissue which has to be aspirated.

Observation (Fig. 5)

Surgeon is trying to remove the cortex and epinucleus near the incision as a starting point.

Irrigation - Aspiration of Epinucleus and Cortex

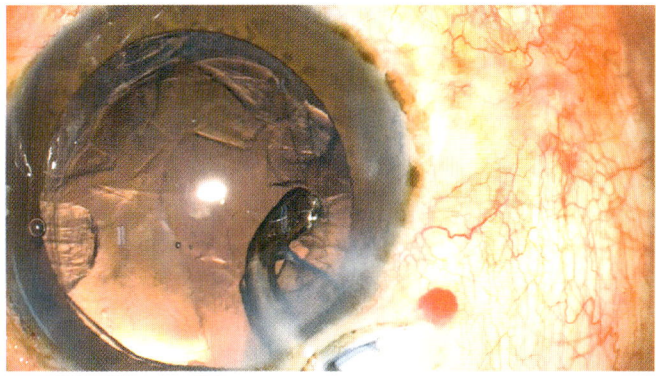

Fig. 5

Results

- Irrigation-aspiration cannula can come out of incision.
- Anterior chamber can get leak.

Do's
Usually irrigation-aspiration should be started away from incision site, it means that from 6 o'clock, then mid zone, and lastly near the incision site.

Observation (Figs. 6A and B)

Small chunk of nucleus and thread-like debris seen at aspiration port.

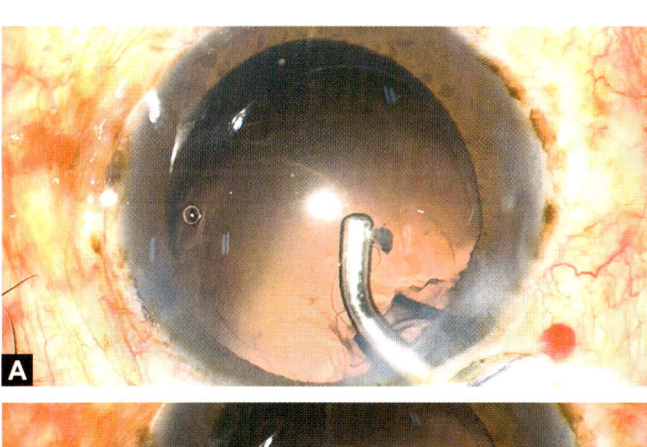

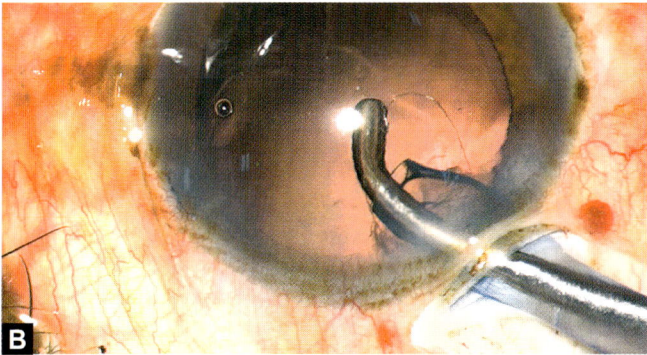

Figs. 6A and B

Result

Aspiration port of cannula can get blocked.

> **Do's**
> - In this situation aspiration is difficult.
> - Small piece of nucleus may block aspiration port.
> - Flushing of the irrigation-aspiration cannula has to be done which is generally difficult, if nuclear piece blocks the cannula.
> - Sometimes sharp needle is needed to clear the opening of distal end of tip.
> - It is generally better to remove the small piece of nucleus by visco expression.
> - Aspiration of this thread-like structure may hamper functioning of irrigation-aspiration.

Observation (Fig. 7)

Shadow of drape is seen on eyeball.

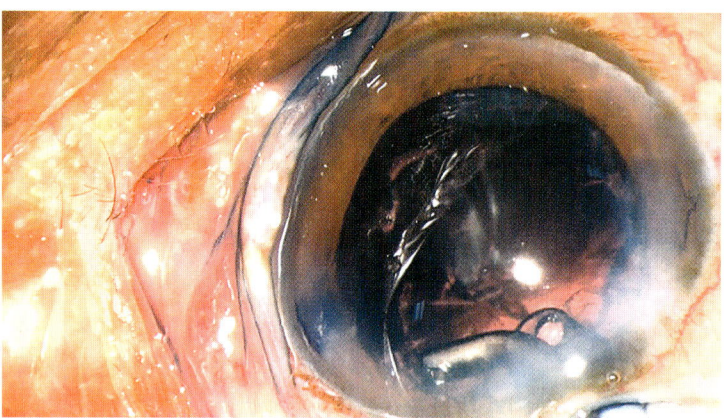

Fig. 7

Result

Visualization is hampered due to shadow of drape on eyeball.

> **Do's**
> Draping should be perfect before start of phaco surgery.

Observation (Figs. 8A and B)

Surgeon is aspirating four fibers of soft tissue.

Irrigation - Aspiration of Epinucleus and Cortex

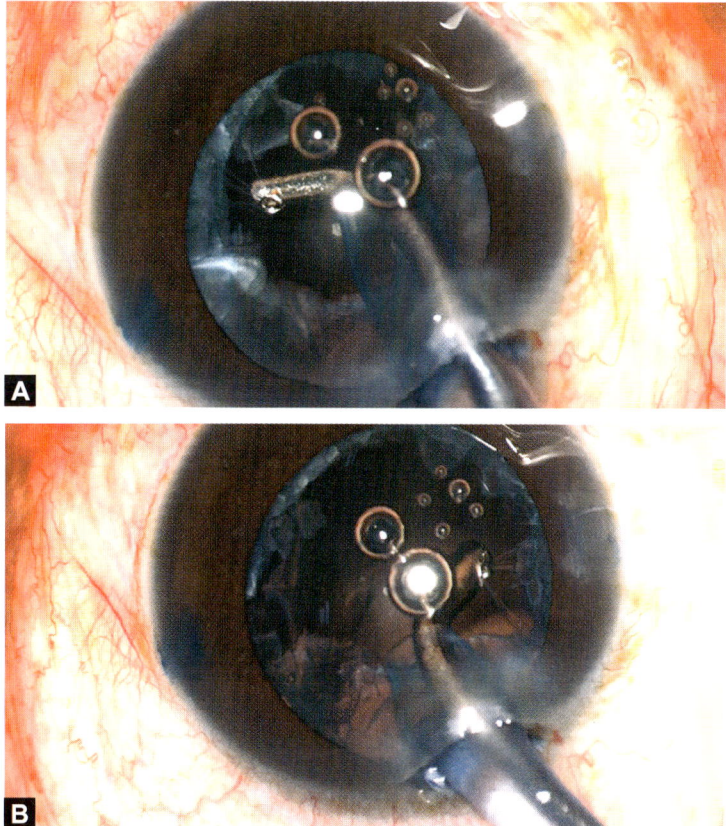

Figs. 8A and B

Result

Stretching of fibers can pull zonules.

Do's
- This situation occurs as aspiration port is not placed in the correct plane of soft tissue.
- Irrigation-aspiration port should be near the bulk of tissue.

Observation (Figs. 9A and B)

Aspiration port is not visualized and it hides behind the iris.

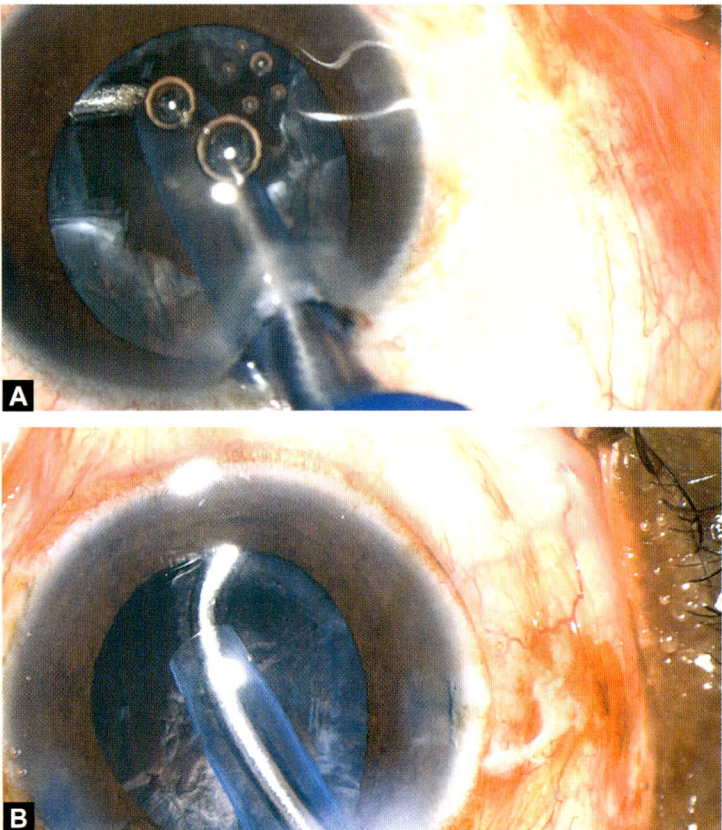

Figs. 9A and B

Results

- It may catch iris and pupil gets constricted.
- Sometimes surgeon can pull zonules.

Do's
Generally one should always visualize opening of the aspiration port.

Observation (Fig. 10)

Surgeon is aspirating over the epinucleus.

Irrigation - Aspiration of Epinucleus and Cortex

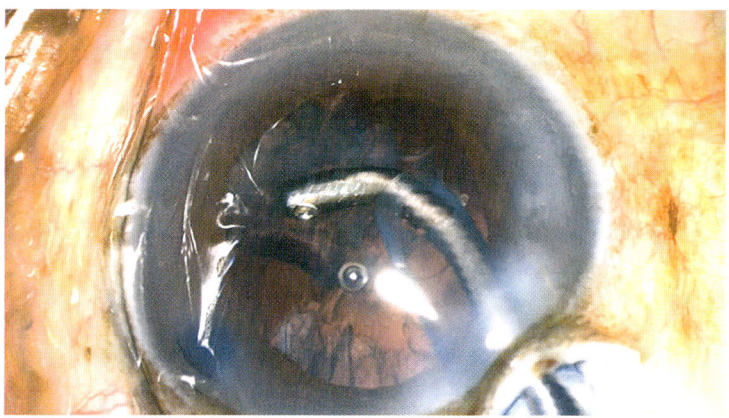

Fig. 10

Result

Pull on zonules can occur.

Do's
Aspiration should be always in the plane of tissue.

Observation (Figs. 11A to F)

- Surgeon is catching posterior capsule as one can see folds of posterior capsule.
- Direction of irrigation-aspiration tip and bag depth is important factor related to catching of capsule.
- During subincisional cortex removal, anterior chamber leaks which is another factor to catch posterior capsule.

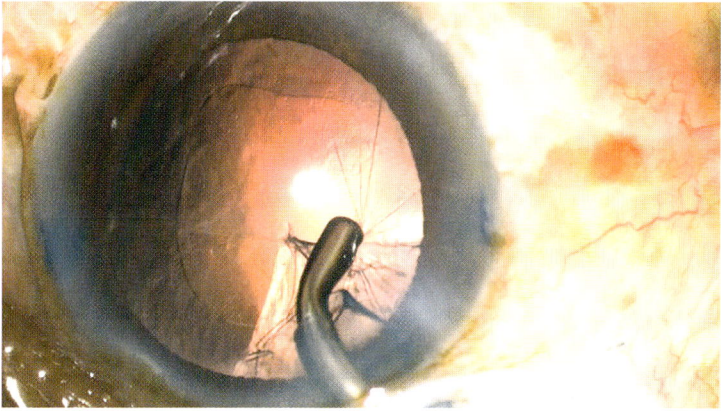

Fig. 11A

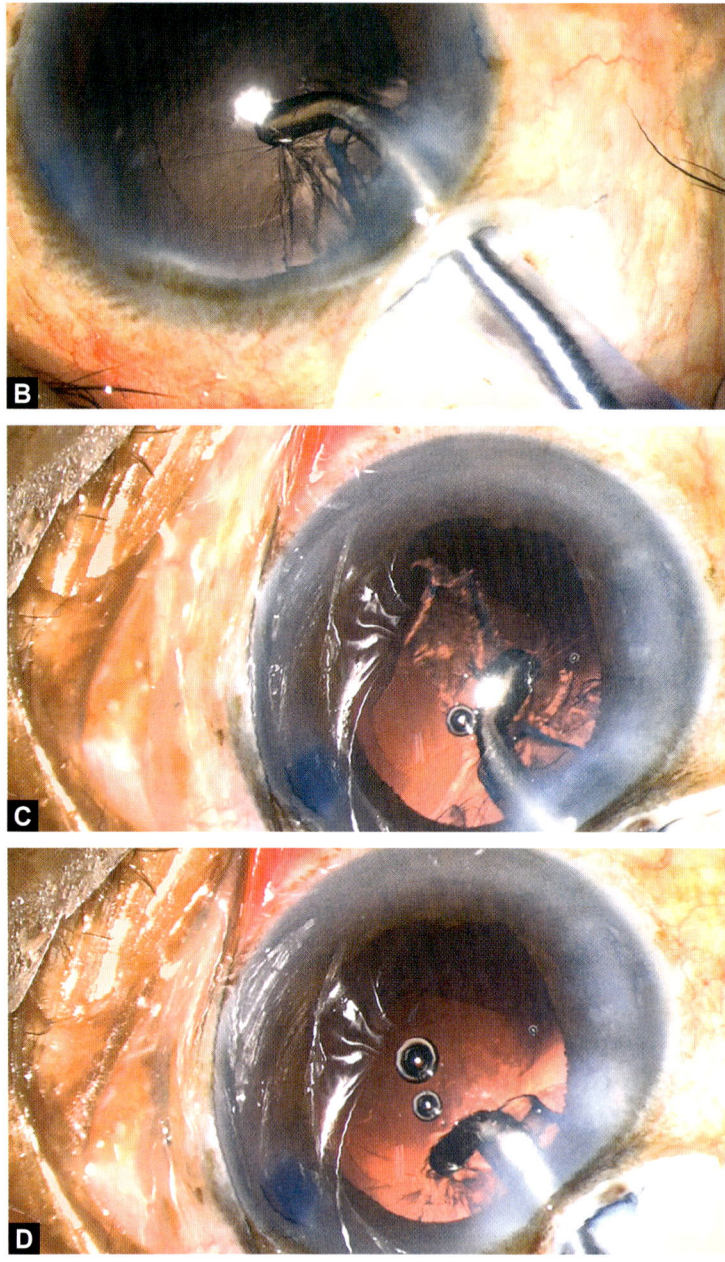

Figs. 11B to D

Irrigation - Aspiration of Epinucleus and Cortex

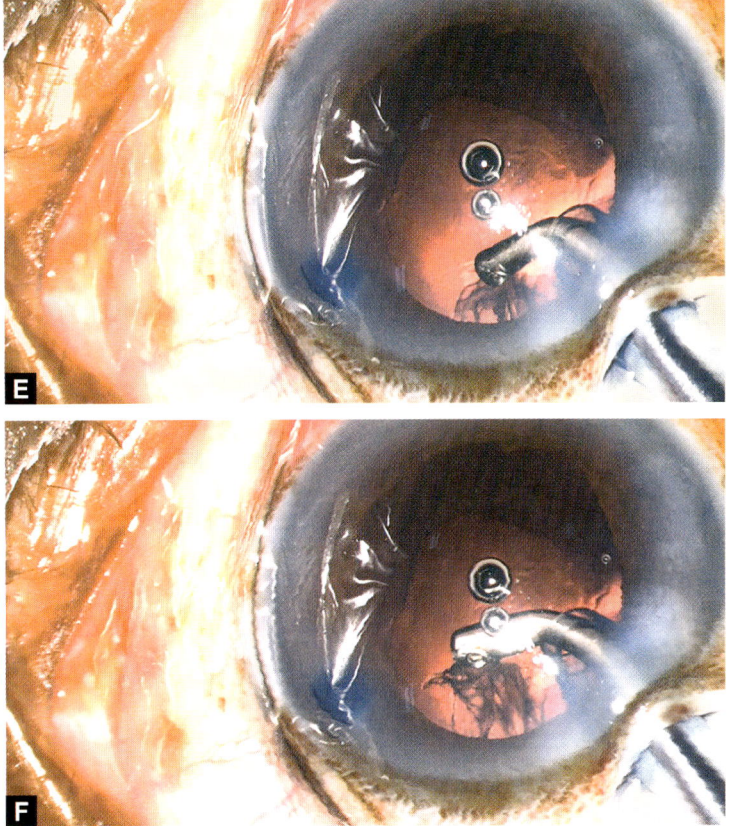

Figs. 11E and F

Results

- Posterior capsule rupture can occur.
- Design of posterior capsule is irregular or very large.
- Sometimes bag can get dislodged.

> ### Do's
> - *Subincisional cortex removal should always be done with better anterior chamber maintenance.*
> - *Direction of irrigation-aspiration cannula should be horizontal or tilted near to horizontal.*
> - *Once posterior capsule is catched, there is tendency of catching posterior capsule with further maneuverer of irrigation-aspiration.*
> - *Removal of subincisional cortex can be done after intraocular lens implantation.*
> - *Try to catch the fibers near subincisional area in vertical position of cannula, and then grab that tissue with horizontal position of tip which moves toward center and then aspirate (Figs. 11E and F).*

SERIES OF PHOTOGRAPHS OF IRRIGATION-ASPIRATION FROM ONE CASE ONLY

Observation (Fig. 12A)

Irrigation-aspiration port is catching soft tissue from multiple points.

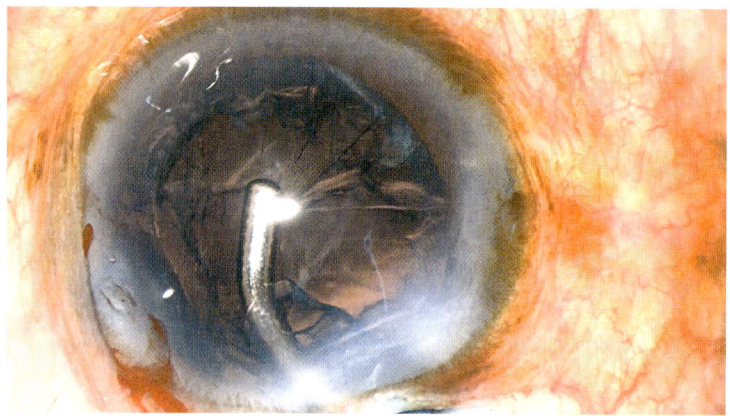

Fig. 12A

Result

Aspiration port gets blocked and difficulty for procedure.

Do's
One should avoid catching multiple point of soft tissue otherwise aspiration will be difficult.

Observation (Fig. 12B)

Fibers are pulled at center but irrigation-aspiration cannula is over the mass.

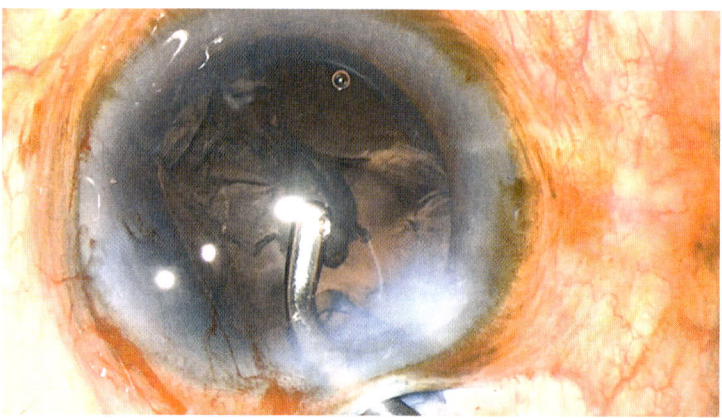

Fig. 12B

Irrigation - Aspiration of Epinucleus and Cortex

Observation (Figs. 12C to F)

Irrigation-aspiration is working over the soft tissue.

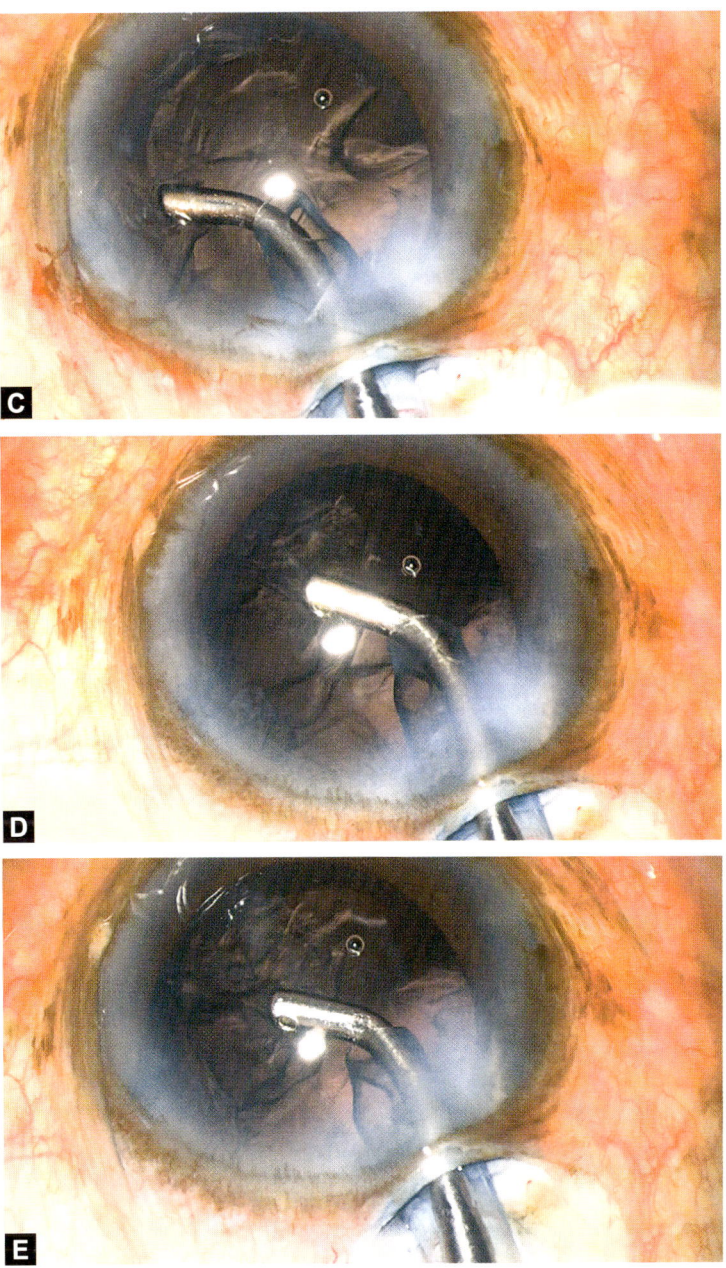

Figs. 12C to E

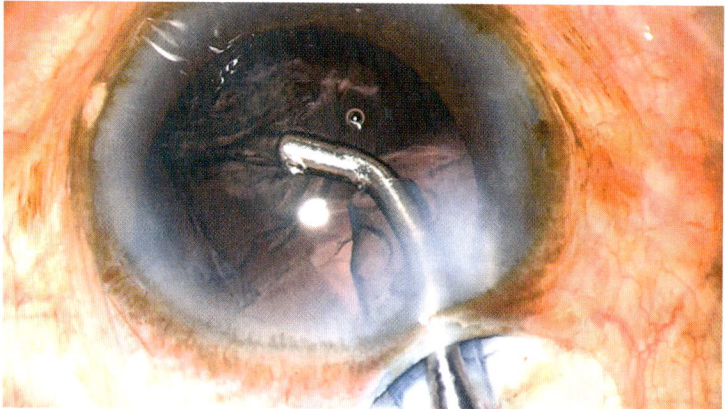

Fig. 12F

Result

Chances of zonular pull and subsequent dialysis can occur.

Do's
- Soft tissue material and aspiration port should be in the same plane.
- Aspiration port should pass posterior to hood of soft tissue.

Observation (Figs. 12G to I)

Epinucleus is not aspirating easily so that surgeon change the position from sideway to bevel-up position to pull these fibers.

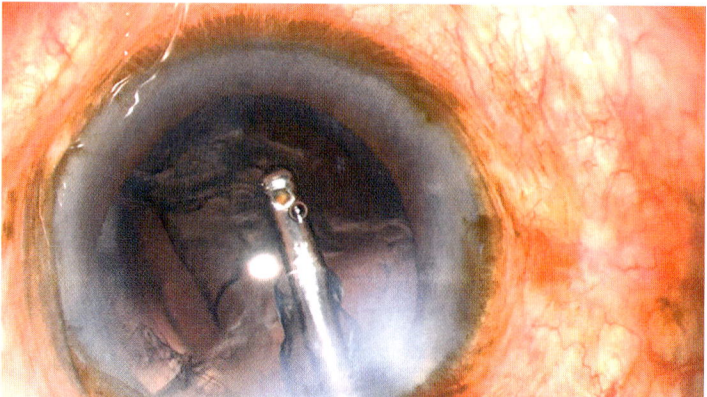

Fig. 12G

Irrigation - Aspiration of Epinucleus and Cortex

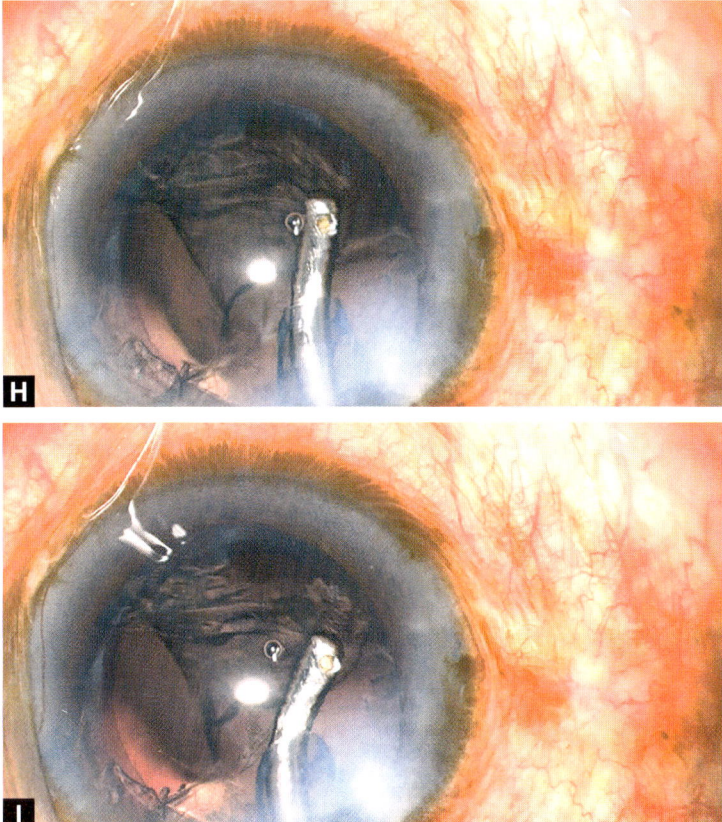

Figs. 12H and I

Result

Descemate membrane can get detached.

> **Do's**
> One should stop aspiration in this position of irrigation-aspiration cannula when moving from one position to other in bevel-up position.

Observation (Figs. 12J to L)

Plane of irrigation-aspiration cannula and epinucleus do not coincide with each other.

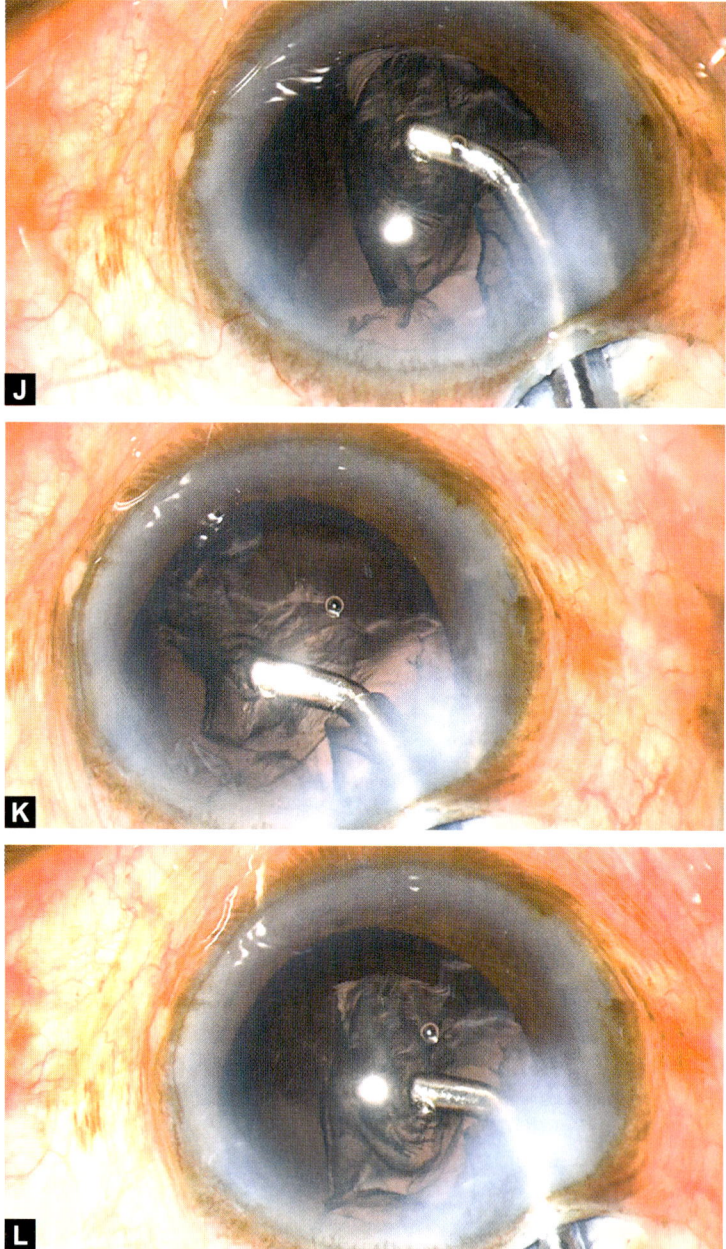

Figs. 12J to L

Result

It takes more time to aspirate this simple mass.

Irrigation - Aspiration of Epinucleus and Cortex

Do's
One should direct aspiration port toward the bulk of soft tissue.

Observation (Figs. 12M and N)

Chopper is introduced to facilitate quick absorption of this epinucleus and cortex.

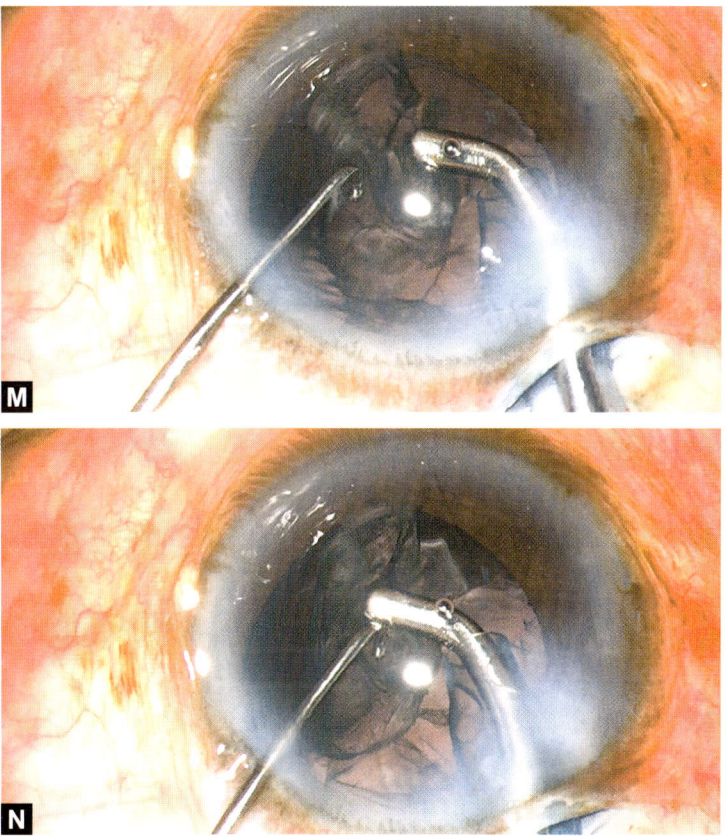

Figs. 12M and N

Result

Direction of chopper is vertically downward which may cause posterior capsule rupture.

Do's
- Keeping the aspiration port in vicinity of soft tissue is important.
- Chopper should pass and work horizontally or obliquely near the aspiration port.
- Tucking of round surface of chopper with respect to aspiration port will facilitate removal of sticky soft tissue.

Observation (Fig. 12O)

Thin strand of fiber pulled toward aspiration port is noticed.

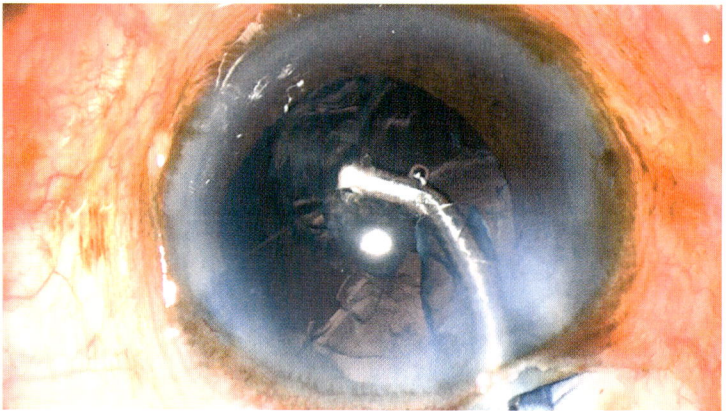

Fig. 12O

Result

Pull of fiber can cause zonular dialysis.

Do's
Aspiration port should be near to bulk of soft tissue which has to be aspirated.

THINGS TO REMEMBER

Port of irrigation-aspiration cannula should be horizontal or obliquely anterior is the proper position to remove epinucleus and cortex.

CHAPTER 9

Intraocular Lens Implantation

INTRODUCTION

- This is the final step of phacoemulsification surgery.
- Result of this step depends on quality of foldable intraocular lens (IOL) and injector system.
- One should do this maneuver slowly and smoothly.
- Plane of incision and capsular bag has to be considered during IOL implantation.

PROCEDURE FOR INTRAOCULAR LENS IMPLANTATION

Observation (Fig. 1)

Pressure of injector system on incision.

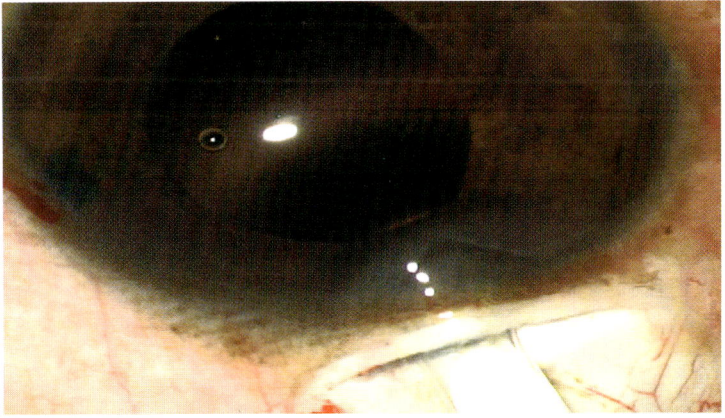

Fig. 1

Result

Incision is distorted during entry of injector.

Do's
Cartridge should be inserted parallel to the iris plane.

Observation (Figs. 2A and B)

Cartridge is pressing the iris.

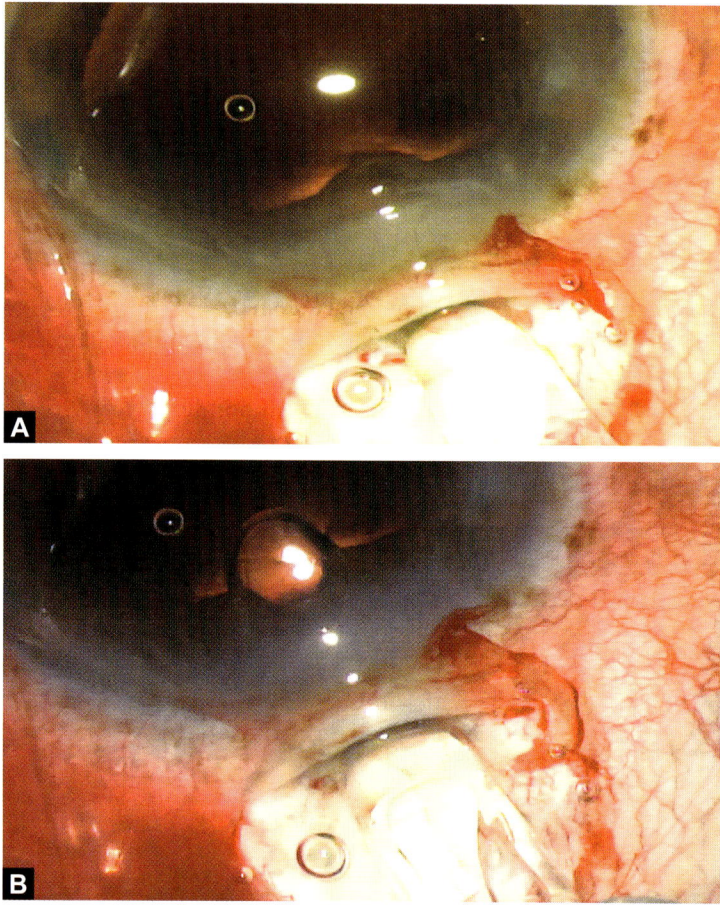

Figs. 2A and B

Result

Cartridge is pressing and pushing the iris which can lead injury to iris.

Do's
- This situation can occur in shallow anterior chamber or deep socket.
- Angulation of the cartridge should be parallel to iris plane.
- Once the cartridge enters through incision, push the plunger to pass the viscoelastic which pushes the iris away for better implantation of IOL.

Observations (Figs. 3A and B)

- Difficulty to pass cartridge through incision.
- Cartridge is going obliquely through incision.
- Folds on cornea are seen due to stretching at incision site.

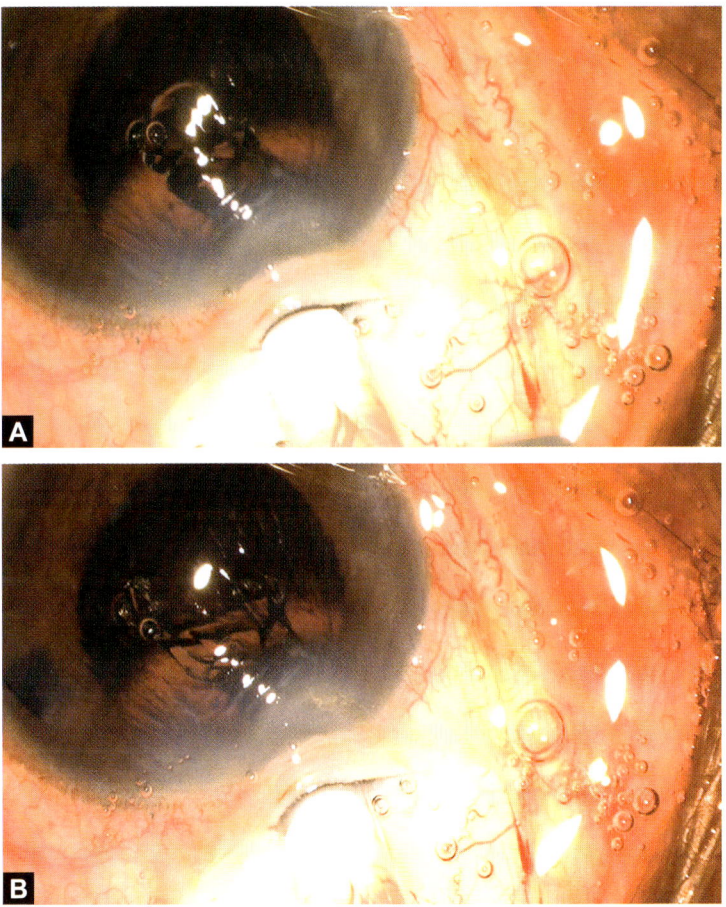

Figs. 3A and B

Results

- Foldable IOL implantation procedure is difficult as visualization is hampered.
- More pressure is needed to pass the cartridge through incision which can cause Descemet's membrane detachment.

Do's
- *Cartridge should pass perpendicular to incision.*
- *Smooth entry of cartridge through incision is crucial factor in foldable IOL implantation procedure.*

Observation (Figs. 4A and B)

Air bubbles are seen during IOL implantation.

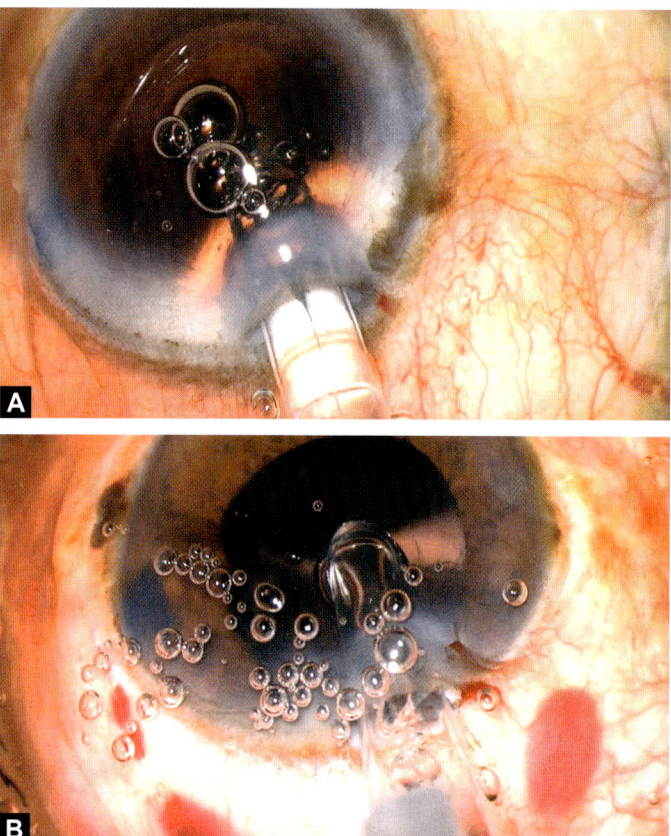

Figs. 4A and B

Result

Air bubbles around the injector system are disturbing the visualization.

> **Do's**
> *Avoid the air bubble during filling of cartridge with viscoelastic solution.*

Observations (Figs. 5A and B)

- Difficulty to pass cartridge through incision.
- This situation can happen due to mismatch between size of incision and cartridge size.
- Round shape of distal end of cartridge can result in this situation.

Intraocular Lens Implantation

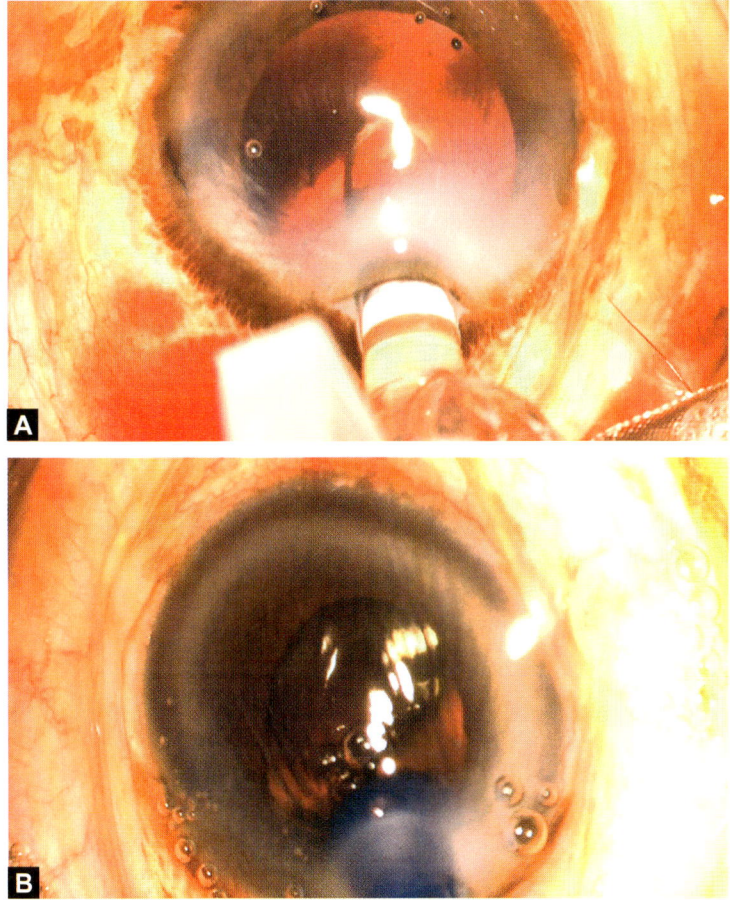

Figs. 5A and B

Result

Descemet's membrane can get damaged.

Do's
- *Use of flat or oval shaped cartridge will be helpful for easy entry of injector system through incision.*
- *Degree of phaco tip (19° or 20°) with appropriate sleeve and keratome size should be proper to avoid mismatch.*

Observation (Figs. 6A and B)

Injector system is reached to the center during insertion of IOL.

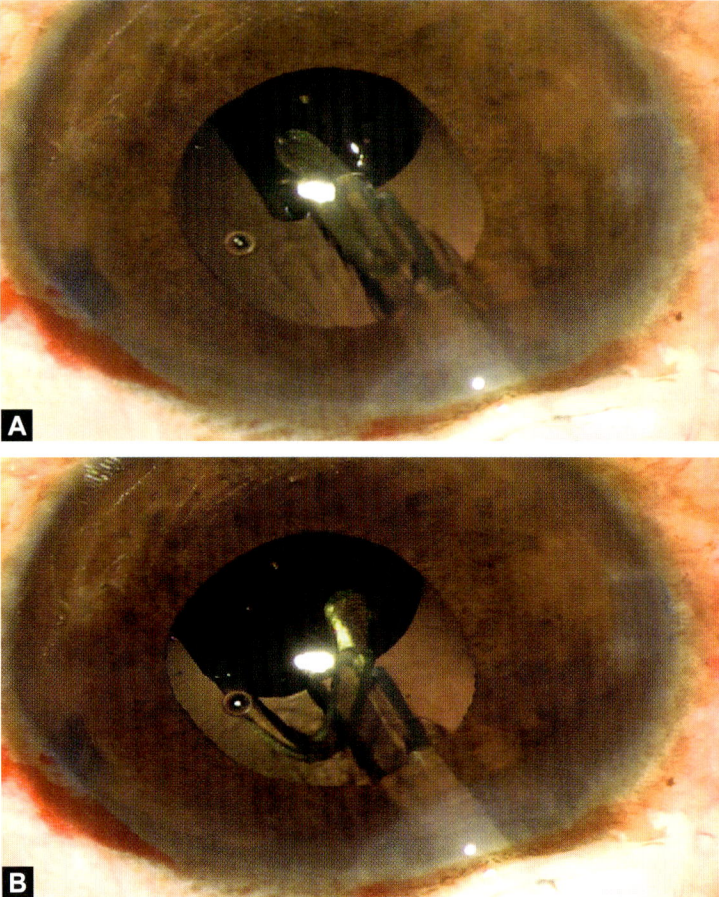

Figs. 6A and B

Result

Intraocular lens can give pressure on zonules.

Do's
- Placement of injector should be near the main incision or just near to capsulorhexis border before insertion of IOL.
- No need to reach up to the center for insertion of IOL.
- Although you reach in the center during insertion of IOL, injector should move back towards main incision.

Intraocular Lens Implantation

Observation (Figs. 7A to D)

Haptic of IOL is stuck at incision site.

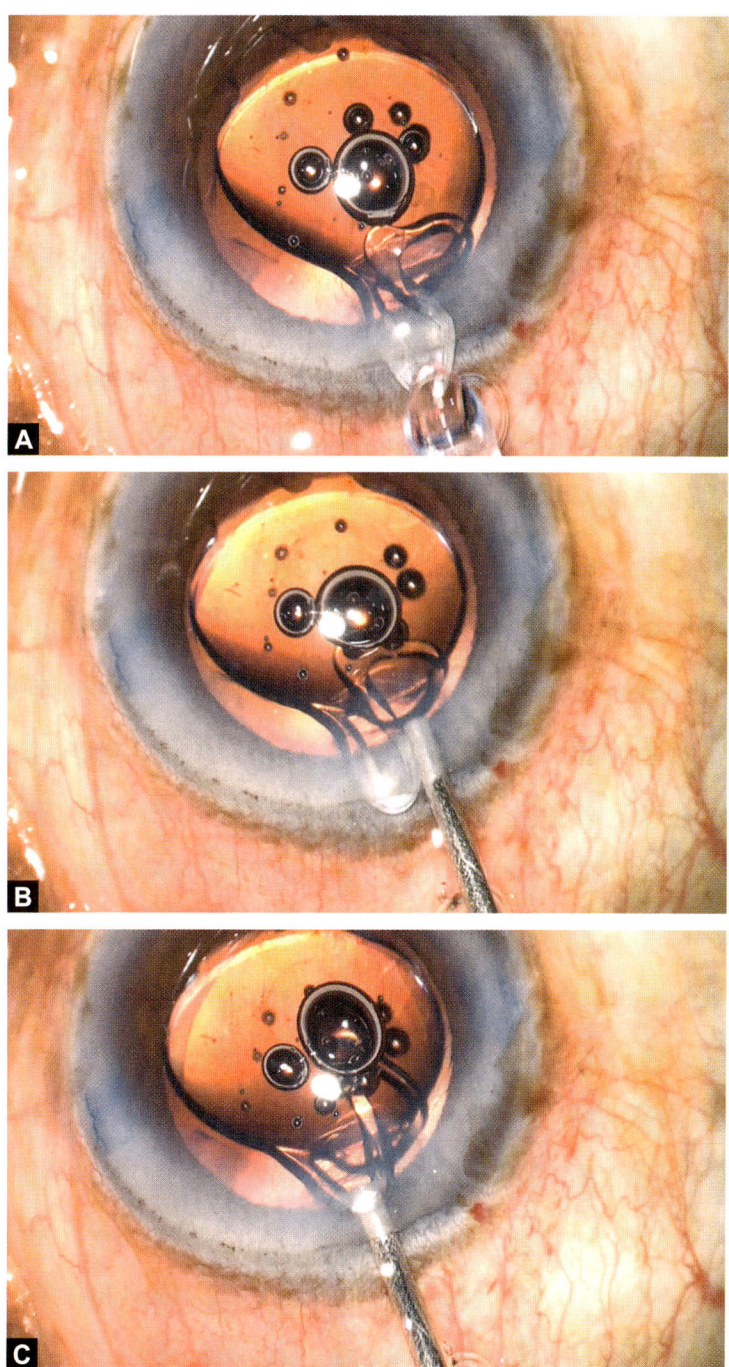

Figs. 7A to C

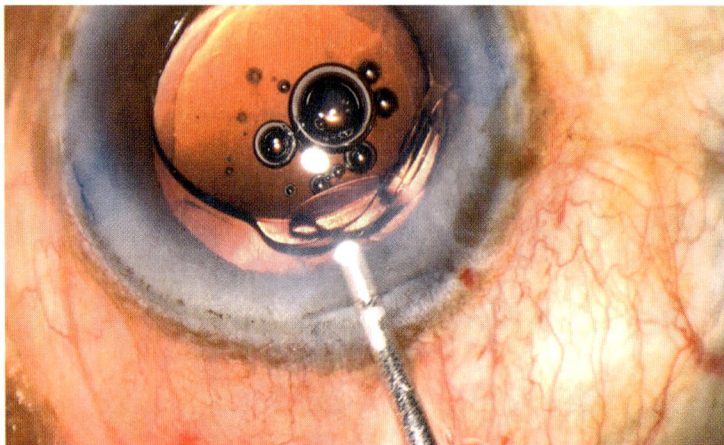

Fig. 7D

Result

Haptic can get damaged or torn.

> **Do's**
> - *Confirm the complete insertion of IOL before removing the injector out of anterior chamber.*
> - *Visco cannula is helping to push the haptic inside through main incision to put the IOL in the bag.*

Observations (Figs. 8A to D)

- Different position or points to put the trailing haptic of hydrophilic IOL in the bag with visco cannula.

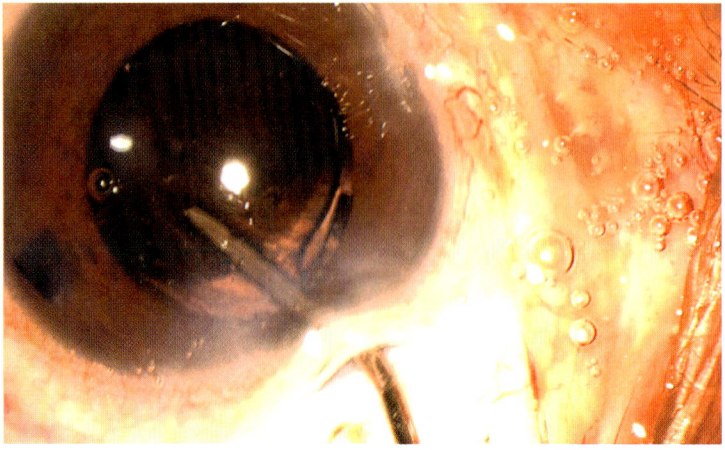

Fig. 8A

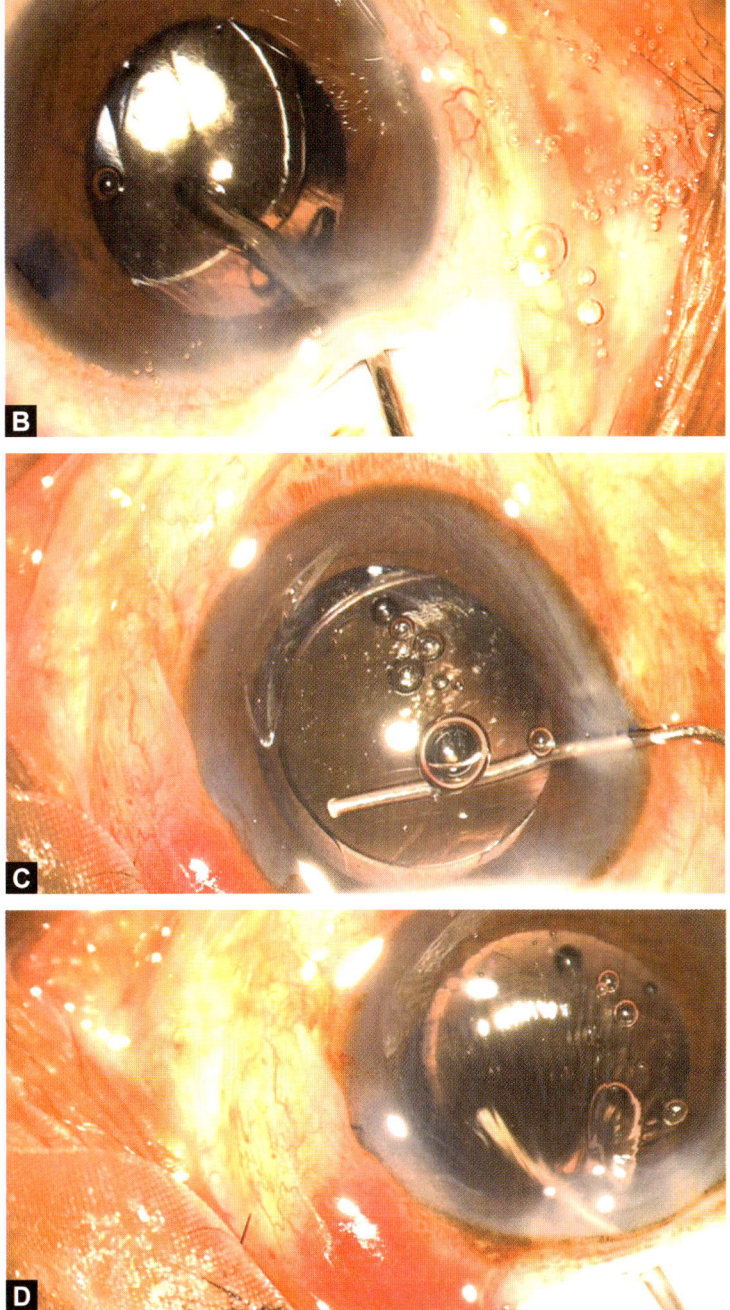

Figs. 8B to D

- Direction of force of visco cannula is parallel to the IOL.
- Excessive pressure and distorted cornea is seen due to wrong angulation and wrong position of visco cannula with respect to IOL.

Result

Odd pressure in a different direction can give pressure on zonules which may result zonular dialysis.

> **Do's**
> - Visco cannula is used to form anterior chamber.
> - Force is applied on optic part, near the optic-haptic junction, and directed perpendicular with respect to IOL.

Observations (Figs. 9A and B)

- Intraocular lens is flipped in opposite direction.
- Intraocular lens shoot out quickly can fall in this way.

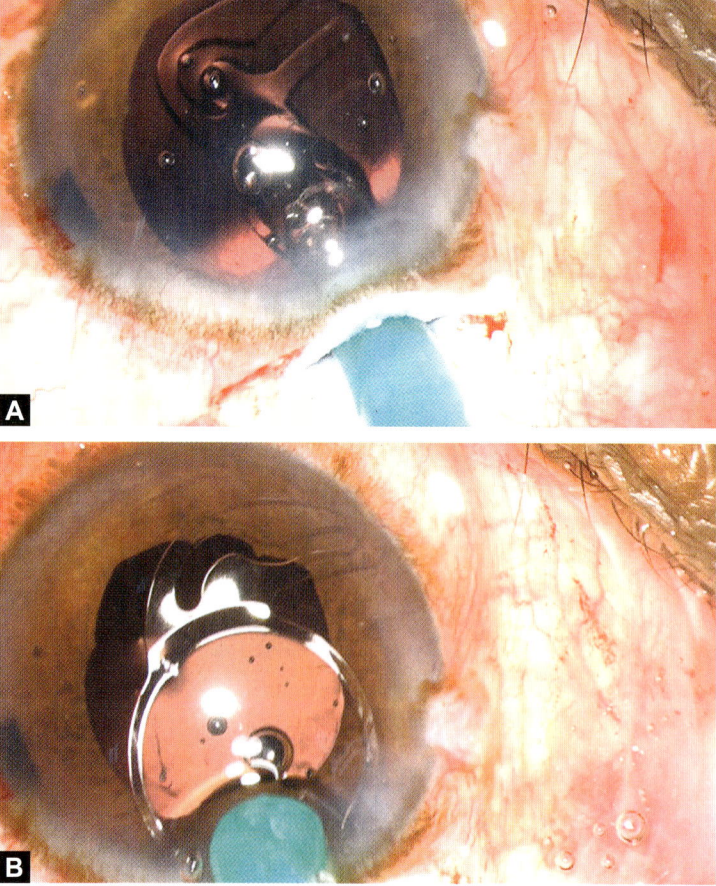

Figs. 9A and B

Intraocular Lens Implantation

Result

Change in refraction can occur.

> ### Do's
> - Intraocular lens should be inserted slowly.
> - Intraocular lens can be turned in opposite direction with the help of high viscoelastics, visco cannula, micro lens holding forcep or McPherson forcep and dialer.

Observations (Figs. 10A to D)

- Surgeon is trying to put the hydrophilic IOL in the bag by pressing or pushing optic or haptic at 6 o'clock position (inferiorly).
- This site is difficult to manipulate the IOL.

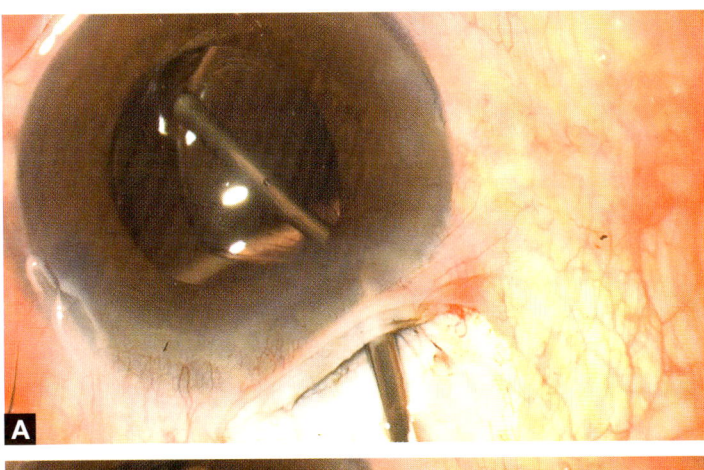

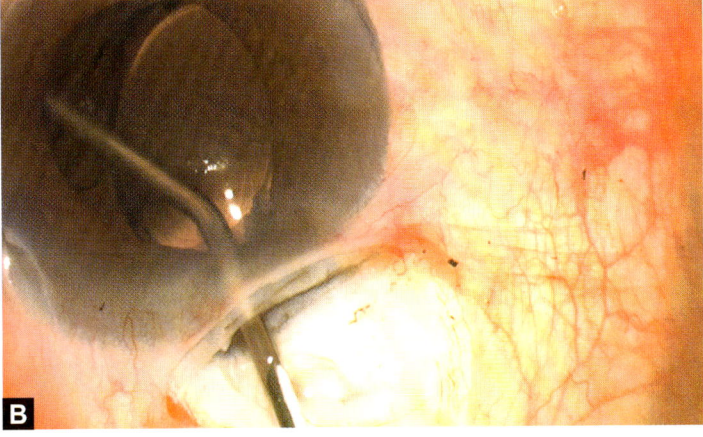

Figs. 10A and B

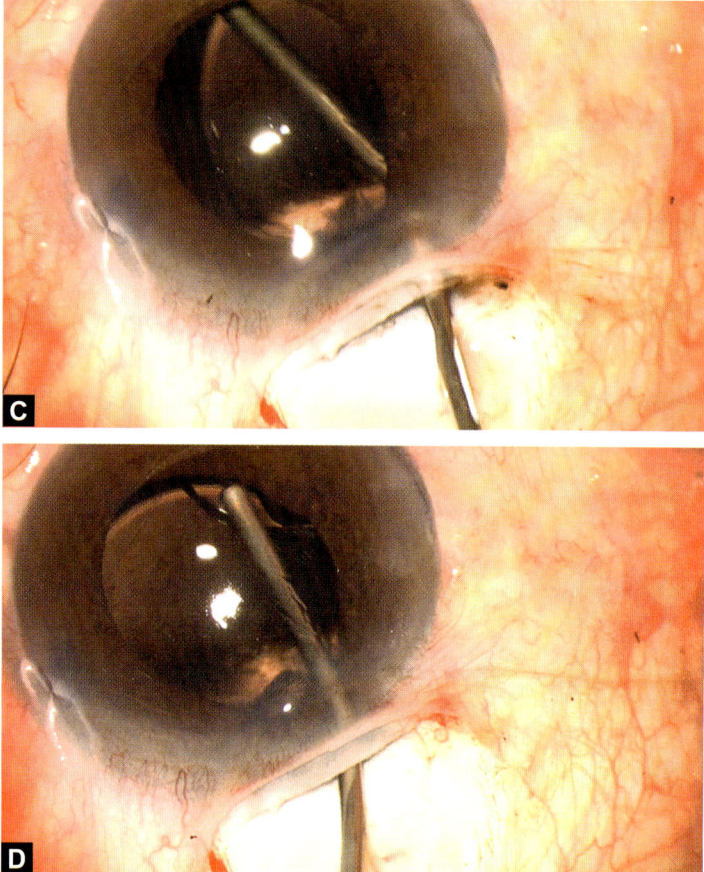

Figs. 10C and D

Result

Pressure on zonules can occur which leads to zonular dialysis.

Do's
- Avoid the pressure on the IOL at 6 o'clock position.
- Try to rotate the IOL and bring the optic-haptic junction superiorly (near incision) and then push it in the bag.

Observations (Figs. 11A to F)

- Visualization of foldable IOL implantation procedure is difficult due to air bubbles.
- IOL placement is not seen clearly.

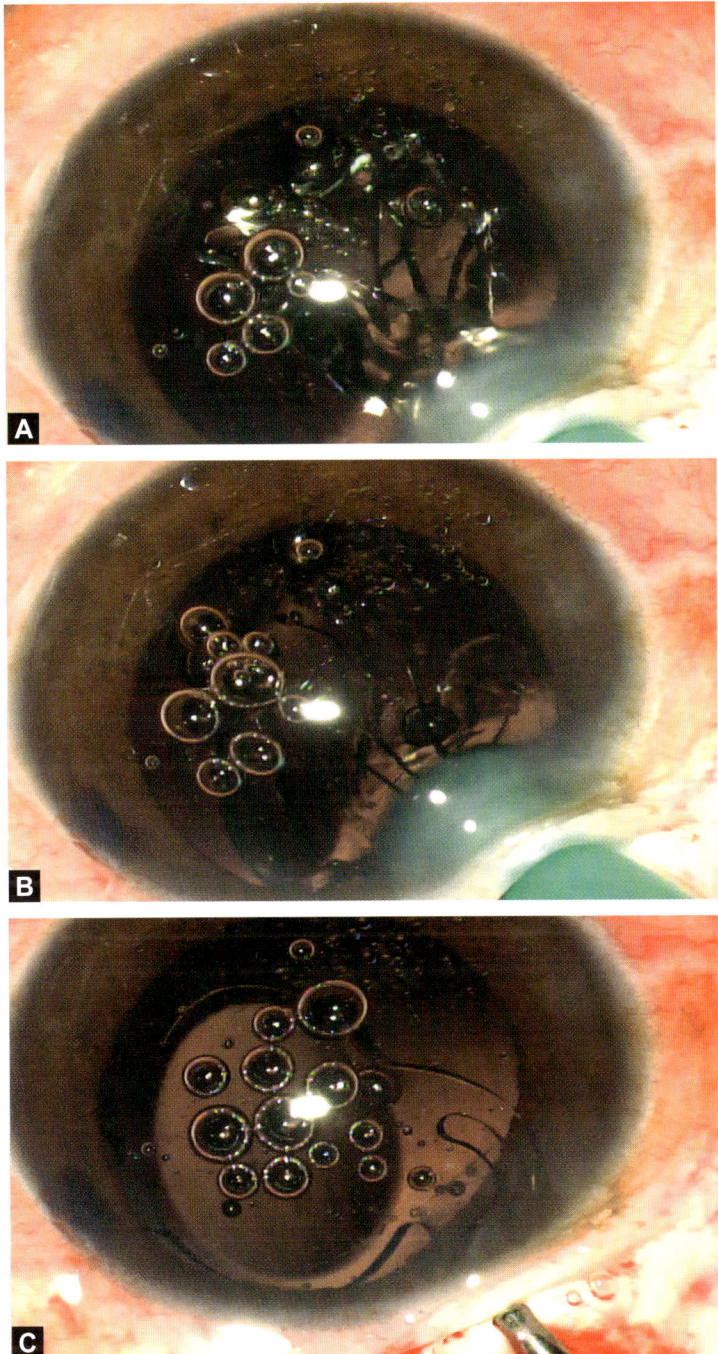

Figs. 11A to C

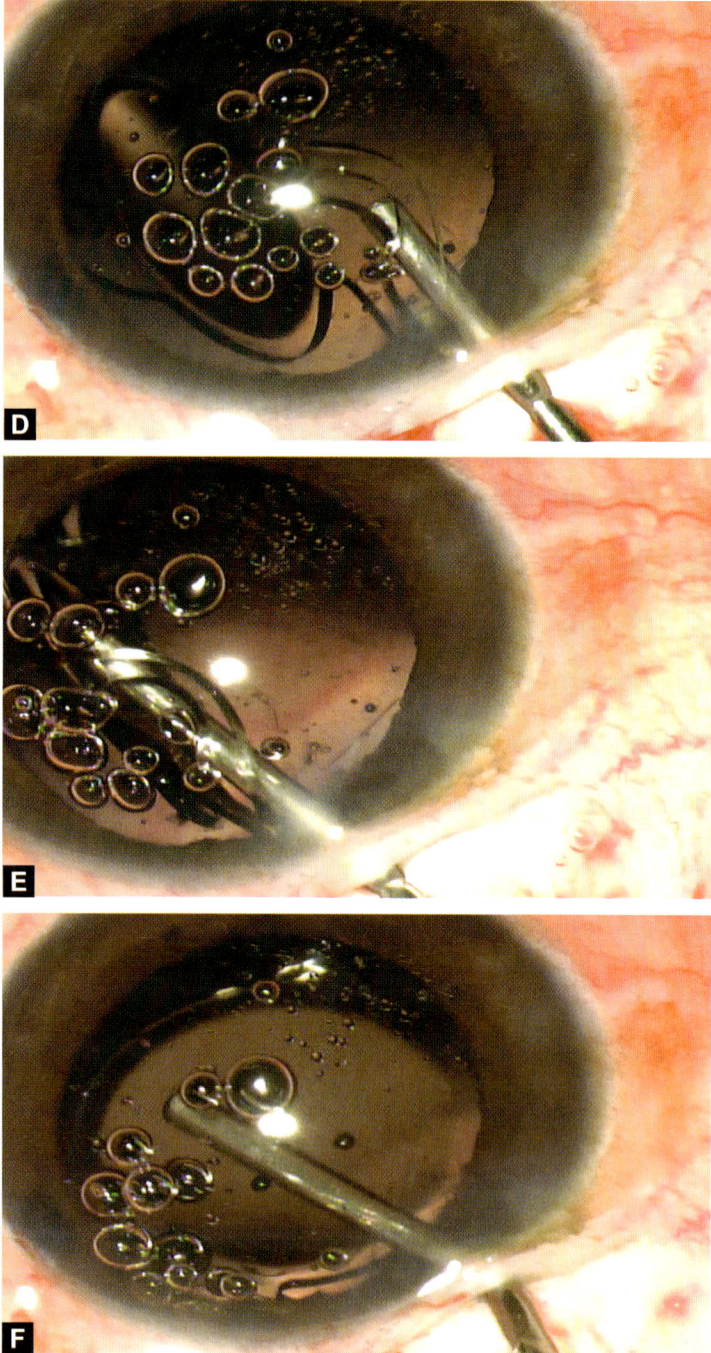

Figs. 11D to F

Result

IOL placed vertically then flipped in opposite direction.

> *Do's*
> - Avoid the air bubbles for better visualization of IOL implantation procedure.
> - Visco cannula is used to turn the position of IOL.

Observation (Figs. 12A and B)

Intraocular lens is placed in vertical position.

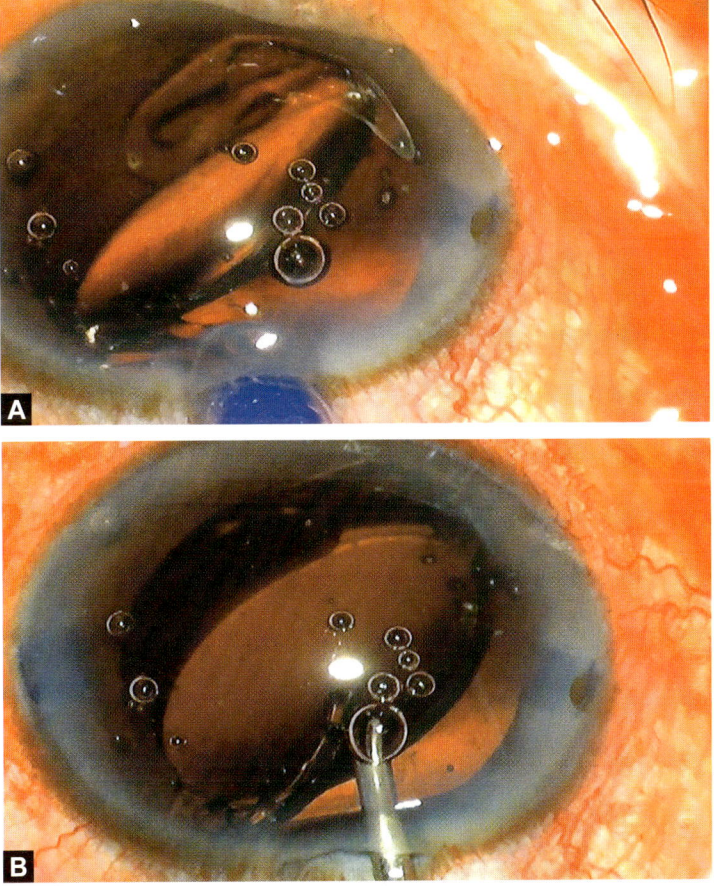

Figs. 12A and B

Results

- This placement of IOL is commonly seen in deep anterior chamber or deep capsular bag, e.g. in high myopia cases.
- Pressure on posterior capsule can cause rupture of capsule or zonular dialysis.

Do's
- *Anatomical consideration of anterior chamber and bag should be in mind which is important before insertion of IOL.*
- *Visco cannula is helpful to make position of IOL flat means parallel to capsular plane (quick movement is mandatory).*

Observation (Figs. 13A and B)

Dialer is used for manipulation of IOL.

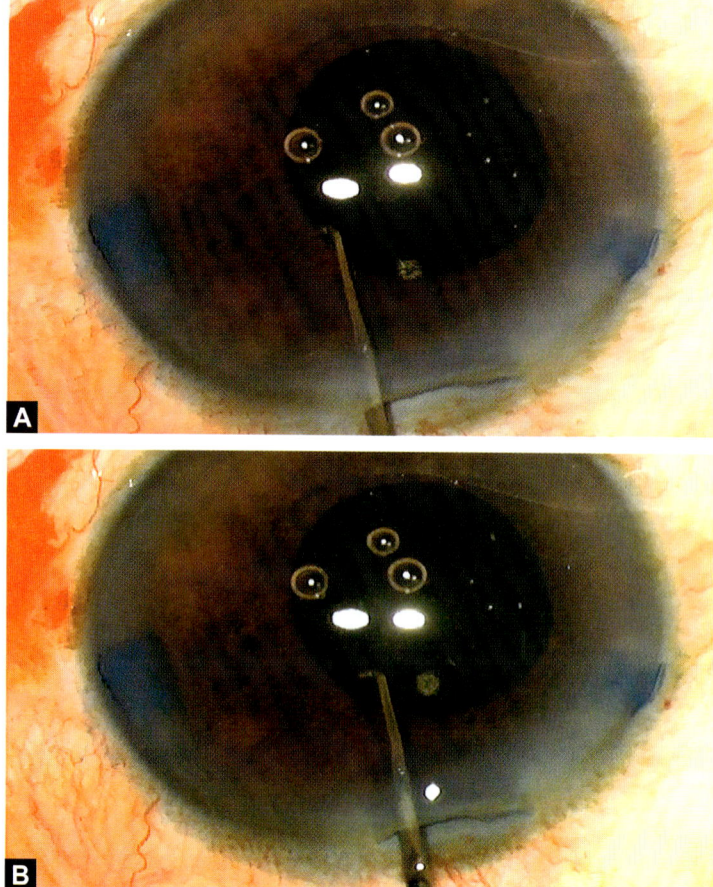

Figs. 13A and B

Result

Dialer can damage IOL, iris, and anterior or posterior capsule.

> **Do's**
> - Avoid excessive manipulation of dialer with respect to IOL.
> - Use of visco cannula is alternative or better option for IOL manipulation.

Observations (Fig. 14)

- Cartridge is noticed torn after IOL implantation.
- This finding is commonly seen during hydrophobic IOL implantation and especially seen in high hypermetropic eyes.

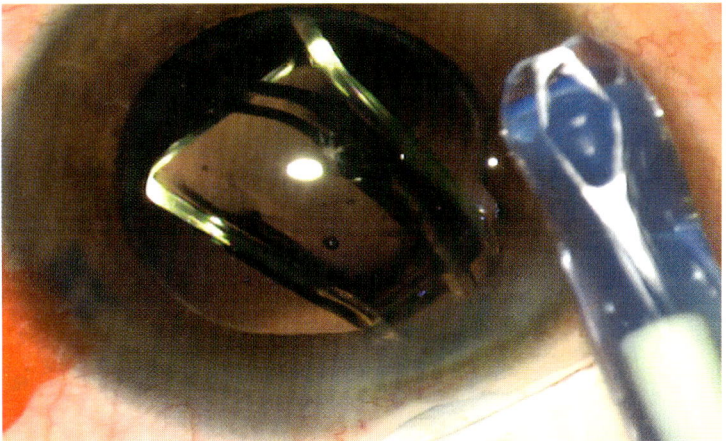

Fig. 14

Result

Intraocular lens implantation is difficult.

> **Do's**
> Many times, this is due to a manufacturing defect, so get it rectified by IOL company.

CHAPTER 10

Surgical Media Center

INTRODUCTION

Surgical media center (SMC) is a unique software introduced by Johnson & Johnson, USA (earlier AMO).

This is a scientific tool which demonstrates graphical waves of energy, vacuum, and aspiration flow rate.

- Green line denotes aspiration flow rate in cc/min.
- Blue line denotes vacuum in mm of Hg.
- Yellow line denotes energy in percentage.

In this chapter, analysis of nucleus management steps like trench, hold and chop, and removal of small pieces is done with the help of graphics.

This software is helpful to all phaco surgeons to analyze their own work scientifically.

TRENCH

Observations (Figs. 1A and B)

- Groove of trench is noticed.
- Foot pedal is on throughout as aspiration flow rate of 10 cc/min is seen as a continuous line (green line).
- Vacuum is 0 mm Hg as there is no occlusion of nucleus in phaco tip (blue line).
- Energy used is 14% and 29% as seen in Figures 1A and B (yellow line).

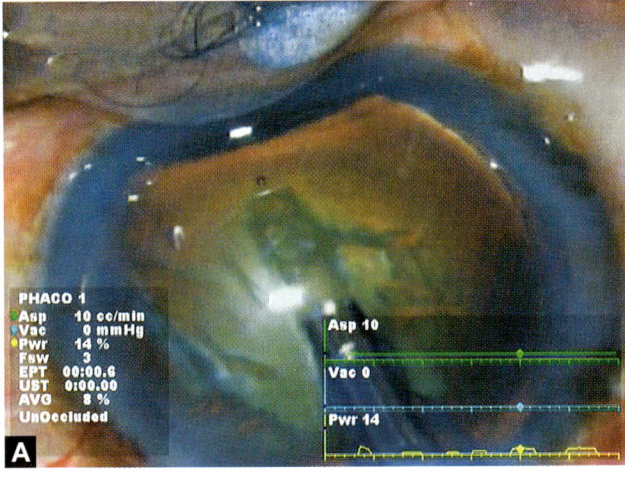
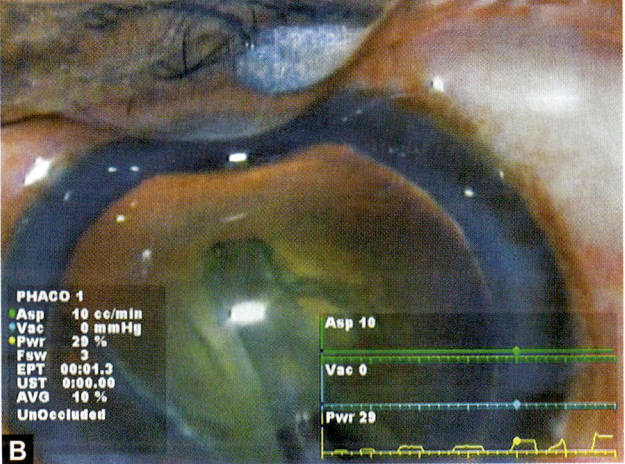

Figs. 1A and B

Result

Energy used is less than adequate in trench which can cause pressure on zonules.

Do's (Figs. 1C to E)
- Adequate energy used 65% which is preset for this case (Fig. 1C).
- Graphs of trench correlate with graphs of aspiration flow rate means foot pedal is on during forward movement and off during backward movement (Figs. 1C to E).
- Energy used 21% at starting point is minimum, which gets maximum, i.e. 65% preset in the center and then minimum energy for periphery (Figs. 1D and E).
- Effective shape of trench should be parallel to posterior capsule.

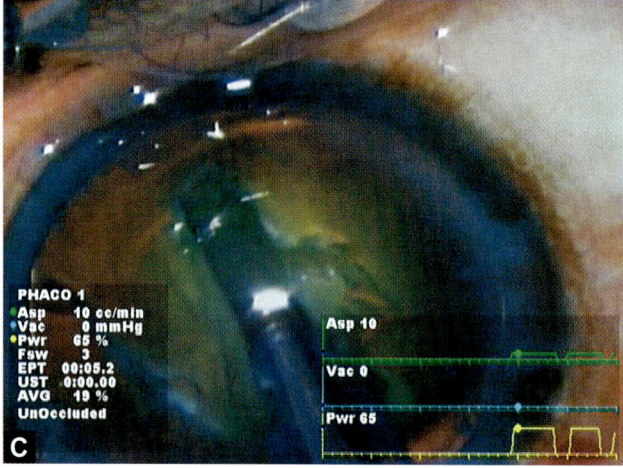

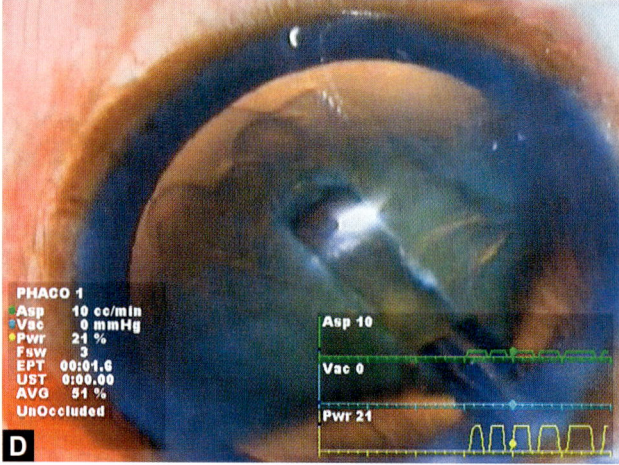

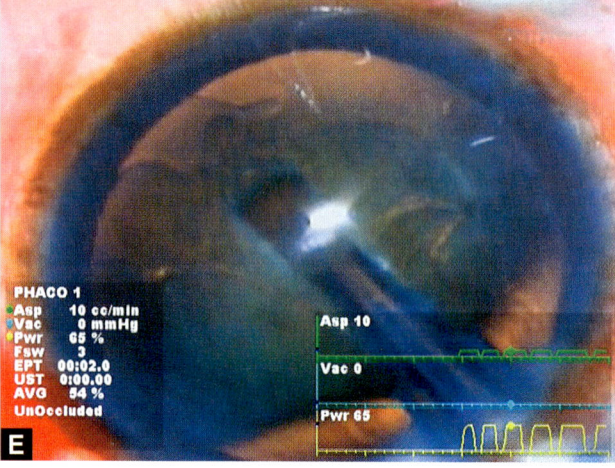

Figs. 1C to E

HOLD AND CHOP

Observations (Figs. 2A to D)

- Adequate energy used to engage nucleus and vacuum builds to preset level (Fig. 2A).
- Half piece of nucleus is pulled out of the bag for chop, but vacuum decreases from 135 mm Hg to 75 mm Hg (Fig. 2B).
- Surgeon has not engaged the nucleus as energy values are seen 0% and same time ready for chop (Figs. 2C and D).
- Flow rate is showing some values which means that piece is still in position to move towards nucleus before vacuum builds (Figs. 2C and D).
- Vacuum is minimum or zero which is unable to hold and chop the nucleus (Figs. 2C and D).

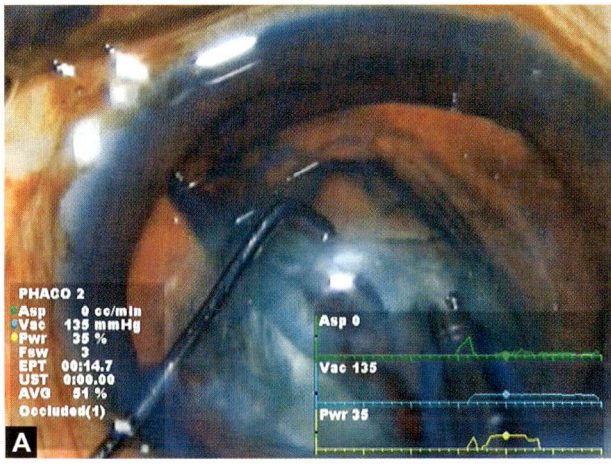

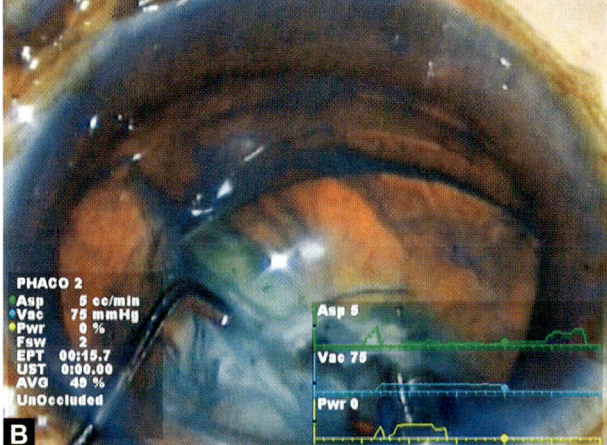

Figs. 2A and B

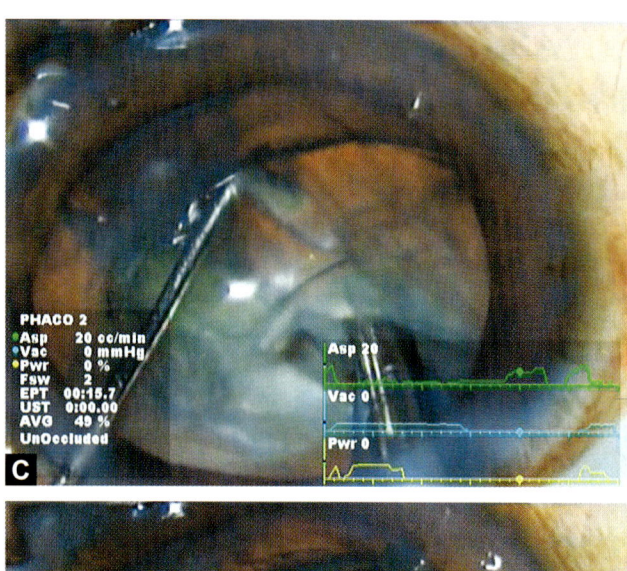
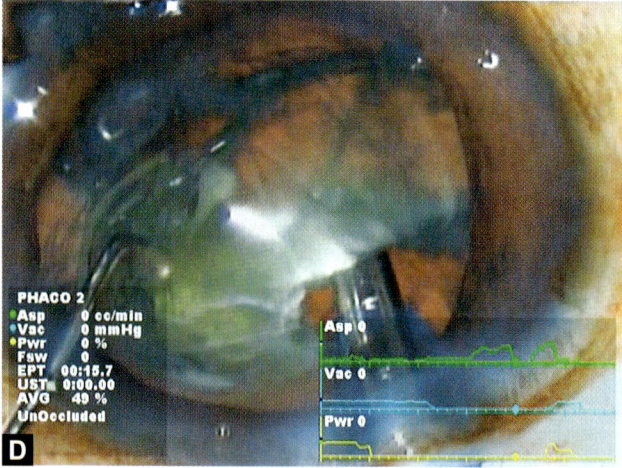
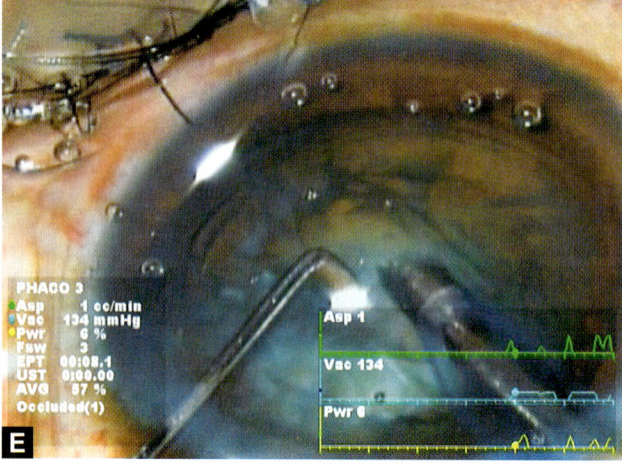

Figs. 2C to E

Surgical Media Center

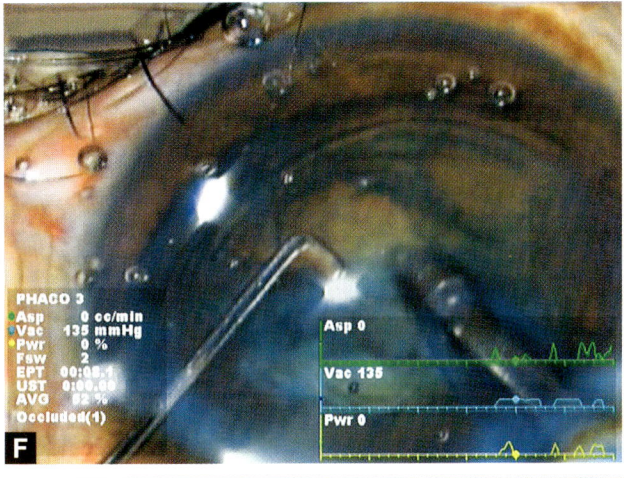

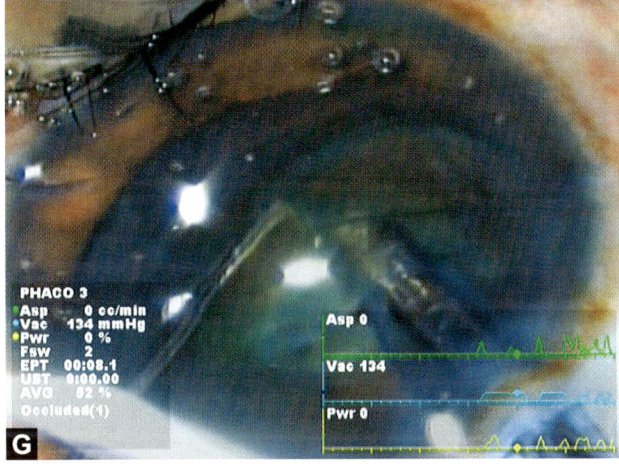

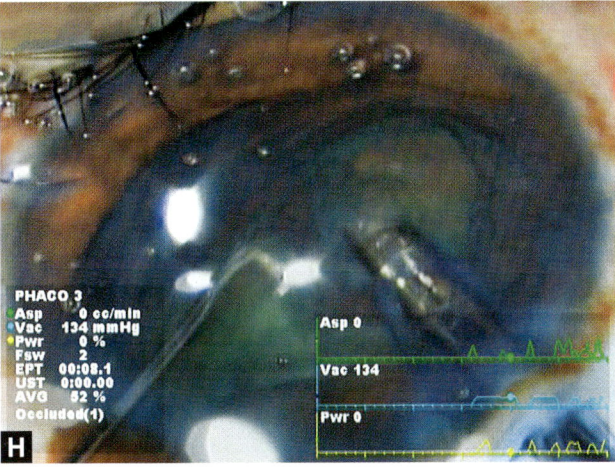

Figs. 2F to H

Result

Surgeon is unable to hold and chop.

Do's (Figs. 2E to H)
- Minimum or adequate energy is needed to engage the piece.
- Hold will occur when vacuum reaches to preset level.
- Flow rate will decrease or reach to zero once vacuum is built completely.
- Once vacuum is built, then hold of nucleus and subsequently chop can occur.

REMOVAL OF SMALL PIECES OF NUCLEUS

Observations (Figs. 3A and B)
- Clinically it looks that removal of piece is going on perfectly.

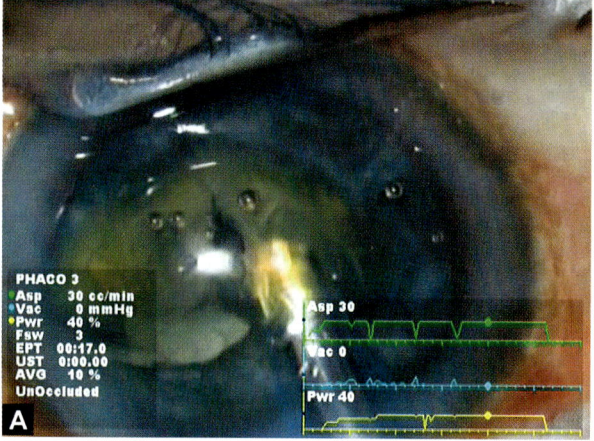

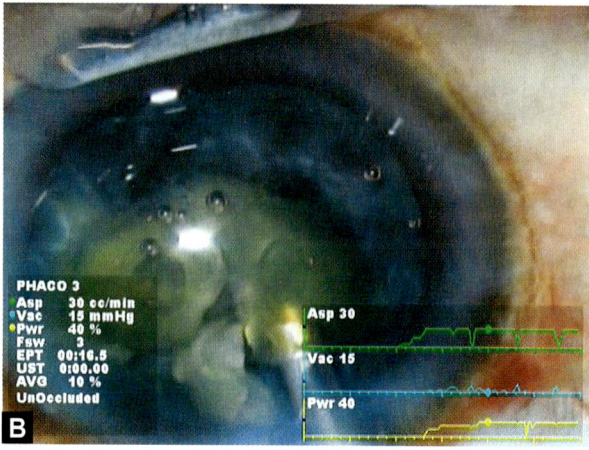

Figs. 3A and B

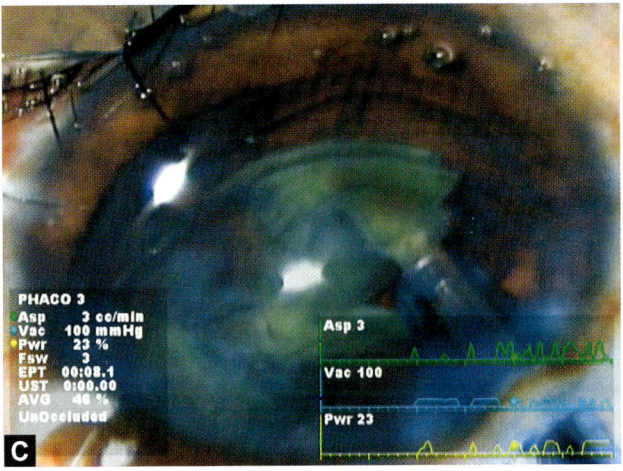
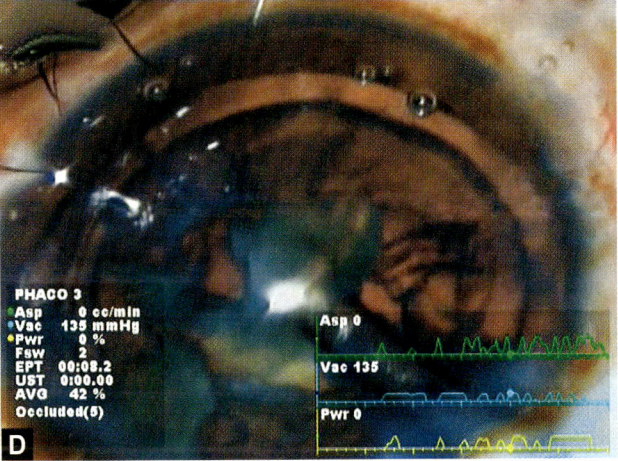

Figs. 3C and D

- Aspiration flow rate is working and vacuum is zero.
- Energy used is maximum.

Result

In this situation, cornea can get hazy postoperatively, as energy and flow rate is working without vacuum.

Do's (Figs. 3C and D)
- During removal of piece, vacuum, flow rate, and energy should work simultaneously for better effect.
- Flow rate will bring piece towards phaco tip; vacuum will built once piece gets occluded and then surgeon is allowed to use adequate energy to emulsify piece.

Index

A

Air bubble 56, 147, 166
    removal of 57
Anterior chamber 148, 149, 178

B

Bimanual irrigation-aspiration
        cannulas 145
Blunt instrument, use of 4

C

Cannula 49
    aspiration port of 150
    distal end of 46
    hitting iris 17
    tip of 16
Capsular bag 145, 163
Capsule 31
    anterior 23, 32
    center 33
    edge of 30, 40
    important 23
    injury to 2
    open 30
    touching of 23
Capsulorhexis 15, 23, 33, 37, 38, 39, 43
Capsulorhexis 5
    controlled 43
    feel of 15
    in one case 41
    needle and forcep 24
    preparation for 15
    procedure 28
    through main port 35
    through side port 28
    Toshniwal microcapsulorhexis forcep 26
    Utrata forcep 23
Cartridge 164
Chop near left side port incision 107
Chopper
    acute angulation of 119
    and dialer 72
    correlation of 98
    direction of 69, 108, 109, 161
    free movement of 119
    handling of 98
    placement of 132
    pressure of 141
    round surface of 162
    side port incision 71
    to phaco tip 111
Cornea 2, 3, 32, 62, 74, 76, 132, 134
    burn 56, 58, 61
    chances of injury 108
    folds on 165
    injury to 37, 7, 13, 122
Corneal lamellae with cannula 15
Corneal touch 6
Cortex, remove 148
Crescent 10

D

Descemet's membrane 6, 16, 36, 52, 165, 167, 159
Dialer 173, 178
    and chopper 84, 89, 94
        division by 68
        movement of 69
        superficial 76

E

Energy 181
Epinucleus 152, 158
    and cortex, remove 162
    near incision 148
Eye ball 140, 150
    distorted 119
    hypotony of 6

F

Fibers, stretching of 151
Fluid, irrigation of 53
Foldable intraocular lens 163

H

Haptic of IOL 169
Hardness of nucleus 52
Hold and chop 183
    case series of 114
    different situations 118
Hydrodelamination 44, 49
Hydrodelineation procedure 49
Hydrodissection cannula 44
Hydroprocedures 44, 50
Hyphema 14

I

Incision 1
    edge of 44
    long length of 8
    plane of 163
    quality of 1
    side port 12
Injector system on incision 163
Intraocular lens 8, 168, 172, 173
    implantation 163, 179
        procedure for 163, 177
    manipulation of 178
Iridodialysis 14, 40
Iris 74, 164
    and cornea 74
    hitting of 145
    injury to 14, 18, 40, 109, 164
    prolapse 51
    stucked 143
Irrigating fluid 57
Irrigation-aspiration cannula 147-149
    plane of 159

K

Keratome 1
    direction of 8
    entry visualization of 1
    instruments used 1
    size 167

L

Lens, hard part of 145
Limbal incision 10

M

Mass
    bulk of 106
    vicinity of 117

McPherson forcep 173
Micro lens holding forcep 173
Micro scissors 15
Microcapsulorhexis forcep 33
    help of 43

N

Nuclear mass 133
Nucleus 183
    big mass of 121, 125
    bulk of 142
    central trench of 67
    chop small piece of 122
    deeper plane of 73
    division of 68
    edge of 102
    management 5
        steps of 98, 180
    mass 107, 123, 133
        pulling of 114
        rubbing of 134
    piece 120
        lifting of 102
        orientation of 138
    proper plane of 119
    removal of 131
    round mass of 114, 117
    size of 137
    small pieces of 186
    soft part of 64, 133
    vicinity of 101

O

Onquer technique in nucleus
                management 52

P

Periphery, minimum energy for 181
Phaco
    fluidics 131, 140, 144
        important for 1
    procedure 44
    surgery 5, 10
        crucial step in 68
        important steps in 15
        step of 1
Phaco tip 8, 9, 52, 53, 100, 130, 139
    and chopper 128
        anteroposterior 108
        division by 83

angulation 98
degree of 167
directed downward 133
direction of 127, 135
entry of 54
in hold and chop 98, 104
part of 56
pressure of 140
superficial 100
use of straight 61
Phacoemulsification surgery, final step of 163
Posterior capsule 153
design of 155
rupture 63, 99, 136, 140, 145, 147, 155
Prechopper 78
blade, placement of 80
dividing nucleus 79
Pupil 18, 142
constriction of 47, 55, 145
triangular shape of 136

R

Refraction, change in 173

S

Segal optiks 15
Shallow anterior chamber 77
Shallow trench, case series of 89
Soft cataract 103
Soft tissue 147, 157
fibers of 150
Sticky soft tissue, removal of 162
Subincisional cortex, removal of 155

Sunayana surgicals 15
Surgical media center 180

T

Toshniwal microcapsulorhexis forcep 26
Trench 52, 180
correlate, graphs of 181
effective shape of 181
superficial 80

V

Vacuum 180, 183
and flow rate, understanding of 98
Vannas scissors 15
Visco cannula 38, 145, 178
force of 171
position of 171
Viscoelastic 5, 19, 30
aspiration of 147
mix with trypan blue 19
solution 166

W

Wound, leakage of 140

Z

Zonular dialysis 75, 140, 145, 162, 172, 174
Zonular pull, chances of 158
Zonules pressure on 60, 72, 75, 80